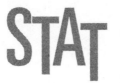

Special
Techniques
in Assertiveness Training

STAT

FOURTH EDITION

Special
Techniques
in Assertiveness Training
for Women in the Health Professions

Melodie Chenevert, RN, MN, MA

Pro-Nurse
Washington, D.C.

Illustrated with soft sculptures by the author

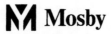 Mosby

St. Louis Baltimore Boston Chicago London Madrid Philadelphia Sydney Toronto

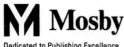

Dedicated to Publishing Excellence

Executive Editor: N. Darlene Como
Assistant Editor: Barbara M. Carroll
Project Manager: Gayle May Morris
Production Editor: Judith Bange
Manufacturing Supervisor: Karen Lewis
Book and Cover Designer: Susan Lane

FOURTH EDITION

Printed in the United States of America
Composition by University Graphics, Inc.
Printing/binding by R.R. Donnelley & Sons Company

Mosby–Year Book, Inc.
11830 Westline Industrial Drive
St. Louis, Missouri 63146

Library of Congress Cataloging in Publication Data

Chenevert, Melodie
    STAT: special techniques in assertiveness training for women in the health profes-
sions / Melodie Chenevert ; illustrated with soft sculptures by the author.—4th ed.
      p. cm.
    Includes bibliographical references (p.   ).
    ISBN 0-8016-7233-3
    1. Women in medicine—Psychology. 2. Assertiveness in women. 3. Assertiveness
training. I. Title. II. Title: Special techniques in assertiveness training for women
in the health professions. III. Title. STAT for women in the health professions.
    [DNLM: 1. Assertiveness. 2. Behavior Therapy. 3. Health Occupations.
4. Women—psychology.   WM 425 C518s 1994]
R692.C43   1994
610.69′6′082—dc20   93-26505
                                                                  CIP

93 94 95 96 97 / 9 8 7 6 5 4 3 2 1

To birds of a feather

Note on the fourth edition

Welcome to the fourth edition of STAT!

A fourth edition! Let's celebrate the "fourth" with a spirit of independence.

Someone gave me a button that read:

"I'm damned if I do.

I'm damned if I don't.

So damn it, I will!"

Assertiveness? Let's do it!

Melodie Chenevert

Preface

Waiting in the checkout line at the dime store, I noticed a variety of tiny booklets covering everything from astrology to dieting to naming a baby. One of them was titled *How to Be Assertive* and sold for 39 cents or three for a dollar.

Feeling amused and curious, I bought one. It proved to be worth just about what I paid for it. I keep it as a graphic illustration of how a valuable tool can be mistaken for a toy.

For a while assertiveness was a national fad. Many people picked it up, played with it, and then dropped it when it didn't become the quick, easy solution for all their problems as some had promised. When it became obvious that assertiveness took more than a few minutes to master, many lost interest.

If there is one lesson I've learned since *STAT: Special Techniques in Assertiveness Training* was first published, it's that, although assertiveness may be cheap, it's not easy. Mastering assertiveness requires a sizable investment in time and effort. Becoming skilled requires study, practice, experimentation, evaluation, more study, and more practice.

Assertiveness was never meant to be an end in itself. It is a means to an end—a tool. Like all tools, its primary functions are to save time, energy, and money.

A tool used by unskilled hands will produce far different results than will the same tool used by skilled hands. In unskilled hands a hammer is merely a blunt instrument. Anyone can buy a hammer, but not everyone can build a house. So it is with assertiveness.

First attempts to use assertiveness are usually clumsy and may do some damage. Remember that in the process of becoming skilled with any tool, you are bound to suffer some cuts and bruises and a lot of swollen thumbs.

At a conference focusing on ethical considerations, a social worker told of the difficulties that arose after she taught assertiveness skills to

clients with terminal illnesses. Although they were often eager learn-
ers, those clients had behavior changes that caused disruptions more
destructive than anyone had ever anticipated. Disturbed and dismayed, she soon abandoned her assertiveness project.

The social worker had severely underestimated the *time* it takes for
the newly assertive person to overcome depression, to work through
the anger that has accumulated for years, and to become skilled
enough to employ assertiveness as a tool instead of a weapon.
Unfortunately, dying people don't have this kind of time.

When asked what she hoped to gain from attending an assertiveness training workshop, one woman wrote, "After this workshop is over,
I hope I leave with the weapon I came for."

Her comment raises important questions. Is assertiveness a weapon
or a tool? Is the assertive person armed or equipped?

Tools are constructive implements used to build and repair. When a
tool is used for destructive purposes, it ceases to be a tool and becomes
a weapon. At this point assertion ends and aggression begins.

Passive people are angry people. They are often initially attracted to
assertiveness because of its potential as a weapon. They literally pick
up a bit of assertiveness and flail away. In their unskilled hands
assertiveness may never be more than a blunt instrument.

By learning to say no, women found they could diminish their
depression and discharge their anger. These were monumental gains,
and for some they were enough. Others began to see that there was
much more to assertiveness than just identifying what they didn't want
to do and refusing to do it.

Today women are taking a second or third look at assertiveness and
discovering that it has even greater uses as a tool than it did as a
weapon. Having used assertiveness skills to free time and energy, they
are now investing these commodities in persons and projects of their
own choosing.

Women are more goal oriented than ever before. And when it
comes to achieving goals, assertiveness has no equal.

In our society, men are typically socialized to be assertive, sometimes even aggressive. Nevertheless, there are men who also need help
developing and using assertiveness as a tool. While this book was written specifically for women, the general principles and techniques
described can be used by anyone who needs to learn to stand up and
be more assertive.

As health professionals, we have a collective goal. We want to make safe, sane, humane health care available. Assertiveness may be the most powerful tool we have ever had to help us achieve this goal.

For years, students in the health professions have been taught that preserving human dignity and reducing stress are vital components of patient care. Instructors have discussed at length the health care "team" and have directed many health care workers into the multibillion-dollar-a-year industry that sometimes masquerades as a charitable, nonprofit health service.

As practicing health professionals, these persons have learned that the health care team is a myth and that the service provided often ranges from inadequate to abysmal. They have learned that our health care system can compound existing stress and create new stresses of its own. Patients must deal not only with their health problems but with the side effects of a caregiving system that can strip them of everything from their dignity to their life savings.

Within the health care system, women have been the silent majority. Although we account for between 80 and 85 percent of all health care workers, we rarely have anything to say about the patient care policies of our own hospitals. When it comes to city, state, or federal health care policies, we behave as if we have no voice, no vote.

When feeling angry, discouraged, or depressed about health care conditions, we can easily blame those (predominantly men) who control the system—the politicians, physicians, and administrators. If it were all *their* fault, we then could sit back in righteous indignation. But this situation cannot exist without our consent. And silence is consent.

The time has come to break the vow of silence, to stand up and say, "This is not the way humans should care for other humans. This is not right. This cannot continue." If you are uncomfortable about speaking up to the doctor and sharing your observations and opinions, you need assertiveness training. If you have never thought it strange that women don't write regularly for medical journals whereas male physicians and administrators write regularly for female health journals, then you need assertiveness training.

Since we are seldom asked to share what we are seeing, thinking, and feeling at the patient's bedside, we can hardly expect an invitation to share on a larger scale. We have to take the initiative. Women especially have waited long enough for permission to speak up and to share experiences, observations, and insights with the men who regulate and control caregiving systems. Whenever a patient receives less than satisfactory care, speak up. Whenever a patient is treated in an unkind manner, speak up. By failing to speak up, we condone current practices.

Students and practitioners need to prepare to challenge physicians, administrators, and other health care authorities to provide a system that is responsive and responsible. This book was written to assist in that preparation—whether it occurs in basic courses, advanced seminars, continuing education workshops, or as a self-help effort. Wishes and good intentions are not enough to achieve optimum health care. We have to stop dreaming and start doing something to ensure that this type of health care becomes a reality.

Women have a long tradition of being nonassertive, and women health professionals are no exception. As I gathered information for this book, I found it difficult to round up many positive examples in which a professional woman had been successfully assertive. In groups, in private interviews, and on questionnaires, scores of negative experiences and examples tumbled out. When a woman could recall a positive example, it was obviously so unique and outstanding in her experience that she had savored the event for years and years.

I hope the day is coming when I will write a sequel so loaded with positive examples that I will have to apologize because all the women interviewed will have found it difficult to recall instances in which they did not assert themselves appropriately.

Meanwhile, I would like to thank the many women who shared their experiences with me. Without them this book could not have been written. They join me in the hope that assertiveness may be the answer for women everywhere who want to give without being taken.

I would also like to thank Ralph Johnson and Argus Communications for the splendid photography and the kind permission to use the illustrations beginning Chapters 2 and 4, which had previously been published as posters.

Just remember, some days you need tools. Some days you need weapons. You need your sense of humor every day.

Melodie Chenevert

Contents

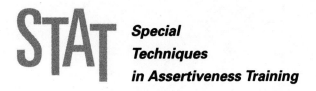

STAT *Special*
Techniques
in Assertiveness Training

1

Of chickens and eagles

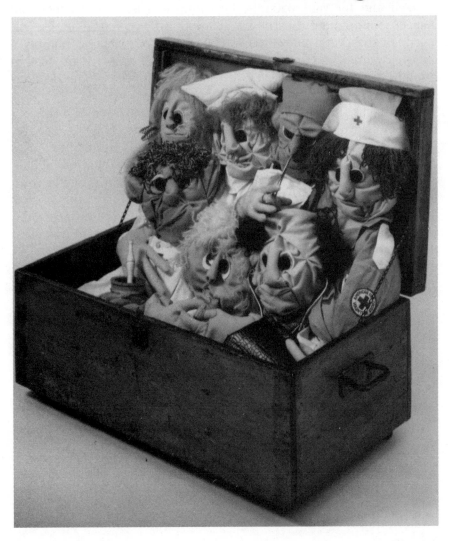

Group health.

S TAT: Special Techniques in Assertiveness Training is a book for women in the health professions: nurses, dietitians, occupational therapists, social workers, x-ray technicians, practical nurses, ward clerks, physical therapists, housekeepers, doctors—anyone female, anyone involved in caring for patients directly or indirectly.

It is a book about learning to be assertive. Learning to stand up for yourself and for your patients. Learning to trust your feelings and respect your opinions. Learning to like yourself.

Although several books are available on assertiveness training, a group of women as large and as strategically placed as we are need to examine assertiveness in light of the special needs our professions place on us.

Women in the health professions have always cared enough, but until now we have never dared enough to stand up for the quality health care our patients deserve. Hundreds of thousands of women are connected with the health care system. What do you think would happen if each of us learned to be assertive? Some think it would be revolutionary. Others think it would be simply revolting.

The question is not "Are you a man or a mouse?" but "Are you a chicken or an eagle?" Before answering that question, read this paraphrase of James Aggrey's "The Parable of the Eagle"*:

> Once upon a time, while walking through the forest, a certain man found a young eagle. He took it home and put it in his barnyard where it soon learned to eat chicken feed and to behave as chickens behave.
>
> One day, a naturalist who was passing by inquired of the owner why it was that an eagle, the king of all birds, should be confined to live in the barnyard with the chickens.
>
> "Since I have given it chicken feed and trained it to be a chicken, it has never learned to fly," replied the owner. "It behaves as chickens behave, so it is no longer an eagle."
>
> "Still," insisted the naturalist, "it has the heart of an eagle and can surely be taught to fly."
>
> After talking it over, the two men agreed to find out whether this was possible. Gently the naturalist took the eagle in his arms and said, "You belong to the sky and not to the earth. Stretch forth your wings and fly."
>
> The eagle, however, was confused; he did not know who he was, and seeing the chickens eating their food, he jumped down to be with them again.

---

*From James, Muriel, and Jongeward, Dorothy: *Born to Win*, Reading, Mass., 1971, Addison-Wesley, pp. 96-97. (Adapted from Rutherfoord, P., editor: *Darkness and Light: An Anthology of African Writing*, London, 1958, The Faith Press.)

Undismayed, the naturalist took the eagle on the following day, up on the roof of the house, and urged him again, saying, "You are an eagle. Stretch forth your wings and fly." But the eagle was afraid of his unknown self and world and jumped down once more for the chicken food.

On the third day the naturalist rose early and took the eagle out of the barnyard to a high mountain. There, he held the king of birds high above him and encouraged him again, saying, "You are an eagle. You belong to the sky as well as to the earth. Stretch forth your wings now, and fly."

The eagle looked around, back towards the barnyard and up to the sky. Still he did not fly. Then the naturalist lifted him straight towards the sun and it happened that the eagle began to tremble, slowly he stretched his wings. At last, with a triumphant cry, he soared away into the heavens.

It may be that the eagle still remembers the chickens with nostalgia; it may even be that he occasionally revisits the barnyard. But as far as anyone knows, he has never returned to lead the life of a chicken. He was an eagle though he had been kept and tamed as a chicken.

According to Webster, eagles are known for their size, strength, gracefulness, keenness of vision, and powers of flight. According to KFC, chickens are known for their taste. Which would you rather be?

The happy fact is that you were born an eagle. We were all born eagles. But if we have the birthright of an eagle, why are so many of us chicken?

Somehow, in the process of growing up, we developed a chicken complex. In our homes, schools, and jobs, we have been kept and tamed as chickens. We eat the chicken feed and lay a few eggs, but the question haunts us: "Is this all there is?"

Most of us chose the health professions because we wanted more than just jobs. We wanted to do something "socially significant," we wanted to be "useful," we wanted to "help" others. But now, job frustrations often outweigh job satisfactions. There are so many inequities. Never enough time to do the important things. Responsibilities are great; rewards are few. When things go well, there is no praise. When things go wrong, everybody is a critic. Personal priorities give way to the demands of countless others.

Assertive behavior may not cure all the ills of the health care system, but it can go a long way in curing the ills of your immediate health care situation. Assertiveness training can give you the skill, courage, and persistence to handle difficult tasks more effectively. You can set your own priorities. You can learn new ways to give and accept praise, as well as criticism. You can deal with people who would rob you of your job satisfaction. You can even salvage your sanity.

You may look longingly at the barnyard and wonder why you care so much, why you work so hard, why you can't just be content to eat chicken feed. Why? Because you are an eagle—not a chicken.

Like the eagle, you belong to the sky, as well as to the earth. Certainly, there are a lot of menial tasks associated with health care. Down-to-earth things, such as beds to make, bedpans to empty, floors to mop, forms to fill out. Routine things. Necessary things.

Then there are those extraordinary moments when the sky's the limit. Moments when you break through and share intimate thoughts, hopes, and fears with the patient. When you're able to meet high-level needs of the mind, the heart, and the spirit. It is the eagle in you that risks genuine caring, openness, and in-depth involvement with others.

Sometimes it seems women in the health professions are afflicted with a People Pleaser Syndrome. We try to juggle touchy technicians, distraught doctors, arrogant administrators, and all sorts of other peeved personnel. Our motto has been "Peace at any price." Unfortunately, the price has often been poor patient care.

Try to remember that you can please all of the people some of the time and some of the people all of the time, but you can't please all of the people all of the time. To live with yourself and to be able to stay in the health professions for a lifetime, there is only one question you have to answer: **Is what I am doing or about to do in the best interest of my patient?**

If a chicken is diseased or has an open sore—that is, shows any sign of vulnerability—the other chickens will peck it to death. We have a lot of that going on in the health professions today. What a waste of time, energy, and talent!

We squabble over whether a 4-year nurse is better than a 3-year nurse, is better than a 2-year nurse, is better than a 1-year nurse. We scramble for status. Is it better to be an occupational therapist or a physical therapist? Who is more important, the housekeeper or the aide? Are doctors better than everyone else?

The question of who is a professional and who is a technician is a visible open sore for many women in the health professions. We each have different jobs to perform. Yet there is really only one job: patient care. The time has come for us to stand together, not for the elevation of our individual professions but for the elevation of patient care.

If there is a distinction to be made, make it between the professional and the amateur. It should not matter whether a person finished high school or finished college. What distinguishes the professional is the ability to do her job with enthusiasm, integrity, skill, grace, and style.

If someone is trying to peck you to death, you can be sure your enemy is not an eagle. At best, it's an old hen or a demented rooster. Your personal and professional lives are filled with turkeys, pigeons, cuckoos, buzzards, ostriches, and albatrosses. *STAT* can help you learn how to deal with all these birds. It can help you claim your birthright and learn how to fly.

Perhaps like the eagle in the story, you are confused . . . you do not know who you are . . . you tremble . . . you are afraid of your unknown self and world. That's not surprising. It is OK to begin slowly. It may take you a year to make it to the flying-chicken level. But from there it's only a short step to becoming a full-fledged eagle. Once you've flown, you can never go back to living the life of a chicken.

It is not a delusion to believe you can fly. It's a delusion to believe you cannot.

Don't be afraid. Come on up. The weather's fine. Stretch forth your wings and fly.

2

Which came first—the chicken or the complex?

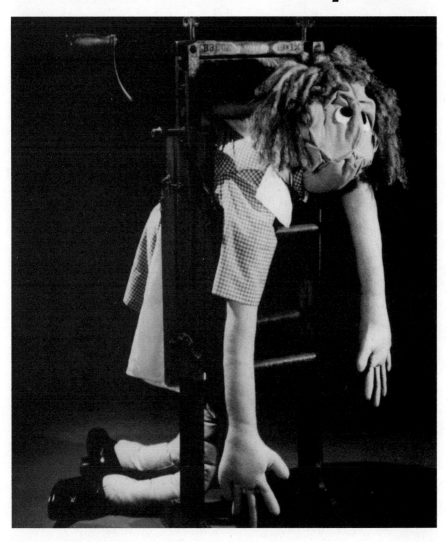

The truth will set you free, but first it will make you miserable.

Before reading further, take a couple of minutes to complete the following exercise. Get a pencil and paper. Now make a list of all the things you like about yourself. If necessary, scribble your list in the margin of the book, but don't cheat yourself by skipping over this exercise. Ready, set, go.

I have used this exercise with one person and with groups of more than a hundred. The reaction is always the same. Everyone is caught off guard. Usually, it is the first time in their lives they've been asked to prepare such a list. They are startled by their discomfort. Why should it be so difficult to write down their strengths, good qualities, things they admire about themselves? They confide that it would be much easier to list things they do *not* like about themselves. They squirm, sigh, giggle. Most find the task difficult. Some find it impossible. That's a sad commentary on our self-esteem. Sad but understandable.

Throughout our lives, the most important people around us (parents, teachers, pastors, sometimes even spouses) focus on our weaknesses, limitations, sins, and shortcomings. Their myopic vision of us is contagious. Keenly aware that we don't quite measure up, we join them in the futile pursuit of perfection (perfection being a rather fuzzy concept whose meaning shifts capriciously with the whim of the person defining it).

From earliest childhood we try to please, to conform, to mold ourselves into perfection. We are continuously measured for perfection against anybody who happens to be in the vicinity—siblings, neighbors, classmates, friends, parishioners. We jockey for favored positions. We struggle to earn the gold star, trophy, plaque, ribbon, honorable mention. We mimic important people around us, adopt their ideas, ideals, hopes, expectations, and plans as our own. They reward us for doing so.

Herded from kindergarten through college, we quickly learn to outguess instructors. Understanding the subject matter is immaterial as long as we can parrot back the right answers to the right questions. Whether our papers are stamped with A-B-C, 1-2-3, or smiling or frowning faces, we all know the markings reflect how near or far we are from perfection. More important, they tell us whether we are more perfect or less perfect than every other Tom, Dick, or Mary.

This compulsion for ranking and rating ourselves against others stays with us a lifetime. Sometimes consciously, sometimes unconsciously, we categorize the people around us:

	Better Than I Am	**Worse Than I Am**
Brainy	☐	☐
Beautiful	☐	☐
Brawny	☐	☐
Talented	☐	☐
Patient	☐	☐
Thrifty	☐	☐
Brave	☐	☐
Clean	☐	☐
Reverent	☐	☐
Other:		
_____	☐	☐
_____	☐	☐
_____	☐	☐
_____	☐	☐
TOTALS	_____	_____

We waste a lot of time mourning our lack of perfection and even more time convincing ourselves that although we may not be better than everybody, we are definitely better than somebody.

The game of "Contrast and Compare" can be vicious. Even though we know it's ridiculous, we've all been sucked into playing games such as "Perfect Mother" or "Perfect Child." Be honest. You remember how it goes! If your baby weighs 10 pounds, hers weighs 11; if yours is bald, hers has ringlets; if yours can say "da-da," hers recites poetry. Nations go to war with less provocation.

I admit that it's wonderful to be perfect. I was perfect . . . once . . . for 30 seconds.

Unfortunately, there is always someone smarter, someone stronger, prettier, neater, cleaner, wealthier, or braver. Someone to remind us that we are not the best. We are not perfect. Of course, we can always point to someone else who is dumber, weaker, homelier, messier, poorer, or more chicken than we are, but that is small consolation. Knowledge that we are not perfect—and the growing realization that we never will be—can make us miserable.

Lack of perfection might be tolerable. After all, nobody's perfect. What is intolerable is the fear that not only are you imperfect, deep down you are not even OK. The NOT OK is a crucial dynamic underlying the chicken complex. To understand the NOT OK, some knowledge of transactional analysis may be helpful.

In the book *I'm OK—You're OK,* Thomas Harris outlines three life positions open to us as children:

1. I'M NOT OK—YOU'RE OK
2. I'M NOT OK—YOU'RE NOT OK
3. I'M OK—YOU'RE NOT OK

Although the first position is no rose garden, the second and third positions are even less desirable. They are generally reserved for schizophrenics and psychopaths. Some say we are locked into our life position by the time we are 2 years old. More conservative estimates give us until the age of 5.

Once the NOT OK is locked into position, it maintains an iron grip on our lives, influencing our feelings, thoughts, and behaviors. It is so powerful that not even 20, 30, 40, or 50 years of additional life experiences can completely break its hold on us.

The NOT OK is a by-product of having been a child. Every person has to start small. There is no way to avoid it. The NOT OK is the mechanism that can make a grown man suddenly feel 2 feet tall or reduce a well-educated, competent woman to tears. It is the muffled voice within that reminds us we are not perfect. It is loudest when we are most vulnerable.

We each have the potential of being blackmailed by our own brains. Our heads are stuffed with 12 billion brain cells, and these cells are capable of recording every moment of our lives. The mind functions as an infinite, inexhaustible piece of recording tape. It begins recording even before birth, and everything that is recorded is permanent. Each moment is stored separately, distinctly, complete with all the colors, smells, sights, sounds, people, places, events, and, most important, feelings that were attached to it. If we could activate the correct brain cell, we could review any given moment in our lives. Think of the possibilities. Perhaps by the time we begin approaching senility, science will have devised a way for us to plug ourselves in and rerun our own favorite memorable moments. That would certainly be more enjoyable than television reruns.

Although no two persons' tapes are exactly alike, there are general categories of information, messages, and impressions that most of us share. These have been designated as the Parent, Adult, and Child. The content of these tapes may be helpful, comforting, unsettling, or devastating. Often their uninvited replay is triggered by circumstances involving tension, criticism, decision making, or crisis. To understand how and why we react to present-day situations as we do, it is important to examine what these tapes have in store for us.

Parent tapes

The Parent tapes are recorded in the first 5 years of life. They contain everything your parents said or did in your presence: all their instructions, preferences, prejudices, warnings, rules, clichés, mannerisms, and moods. Because much is recorded before you have any verbal ability, this content is preserved "as is," without benefit of any editing or qualifying explanations. When replayed, these tapes resound as absolute truth from the all-powerful giants who both nurtured and punished you.

These tapes include some essential lifesaving information on handling everything from matches to traffic. They also contain useful information of the how-to-do-it-yourself variety. However, some bits of information may become distorted and lead to compulsion or rituals in adult life. An example might be the simple instruction to wash your hands after using the toilet. A social worker recalled that when going to the bathroom in the middle of the night as a child, she would be too sleepy to wash her hands and would simply run the water for a moment to appease Mother, who might be listening. She laughs when she shares that, 35 years later and living alone, she still catches herself occasionally running water in the middle of the night to placate the gods.

The Parent tapes house all the words like "no," "don't," "never," "never ever," "should," "ought," "remember," and "I told you so." Listen for them in your conversation.

Child tapes

During the first 5 years of life, the Child tapes are also being recorded. They consist mainly of feelings—gut-level reactions to all the nos, don'ts, oh-my-god gasps, sighs, sour looks, shaking heads, and wagging fingers. Like fossils permanently embedded, here are all the fears of being lost, alone, abandoned, rejected, or disowned. Here, too, are lasting imprints of being tiny, tired, frustrated, stupid, helpless, sad, clumsy, inept, and vulnerable.

This is the price of having started life small. This is the inescapable origin of the NOT OK. The instant replay of the Child tapes can make tears sting your eyes or your face flush with shame or guilt at the most inopportune moments.

Because replay can be so painful, there is a strong tendency to lock out the Child tapes. Sadly enough, when you lock out the Child, you also lock out access to the seeds of creativity, because also housed here are all the warm, happy, carefree, joyful, curiosity-tickling experiences; all the "firsts"; all the "Aha!" feelings connected with exploration and discovery. What toddler hasn't beamed when he discovered the light switch and momentarily held power over light and darkness?

Adult tapes

At about 10 months of age, the Adult begins operating. In contrast to the Parent (taught concept of life) and the Child (felt concept of life), the Adult thinks out its own concept of life. Gathering information through all the senses, the Adult asks questions such as Who? What? Where? When? Why? How? and How much? "How much?" That has to be the least-asked question in health care. Even consumers who are avid comparison shoppers for every other product or service rarely inquire about, let alone quibble over, medical costs.

Years ago when I had to have a vein stripping, I returned to my alma mater in Rochester, Minnesota. An internationally known surgeon at the Mayo Clinic performed the surgery. When the bill came, I was amused to see that his charge for operating room time was $6 per minute. I hadn't realized that was how the price was determined.

Out of curiosity I asked my local physician, who had been miffed by my refusal to let him do the surgery, what his fee per minute was in the operating room. His fee was $8. Sometimes the best care actually costs less.

It is also the Adult's responsibility to weigh possible outcomes, estimate the probabilities of success or failure, and then make decisions. For example, most of us jaywalk occasionally. Standing in the middle of the block eyeing the ice cream parlor on the other side of the street, we are strongly tempted to dash straight across (Child). The Parent interrupts, reminding us to cross only at the intersection on the green light (twinge of guilt). The Adult takes over and begins estimating probabilities of such things as our being caught by a policeman (Parent) or of our being run over by a Greyhound bus. After gathering, sorting, and evaluating the information, the Adult decides whether we jaywalk, cross at the intersection, or go home without ice cream.

Another important function of the Adult is to update the information and impressions stored in the Parent and Child, making them relevant and reliable. If the Parent is too threatening or restrictive, the Adult may shy away from correcting those tapes and literally follow in Mother's or Father's footsteps. The Adult is then said to be *contaminated* by the Parent. If the Parent tapes are incomplete or inaudible, the Adult may be ruled by the Child, and a carefree, impulsive, irresponsible person may be the result.

•　　　•　　　•

When talking with another person (doctor, patient, employer, or spouse), listen for the Parent or Child to intrude. If you have the urge to take over, lecture, scold, threaten, or dictate how things should be, your Parent is in control. On the other hand, if you have the urge to cry, scream, giggle, obey, or hide, your Child is in control. Slips from Adult into Parent or Child are common and normal. Sometimes they are helpful, sometimes harmful. You can develop the sensitivity necessary to assess how appropriate your responses are in each situation.

The mature person has comfortable access to all three and is able to use each component to advantage. The Parent keeps the mind uncluttered by making mundane decisions automatically and supplying useful information. The Child provides the exuberance, humor, and imagination necessary for creative problem solving and innovative living. The Adult continuously gathers, sifts, sorts, and stores information while determining the present course of action.

For the person struggling with assertiveness, a group experience in transactional analysis may be just as helpful as an assertiveness training group. Assertiveness depends on your ability to stay in the Adult. That means being able to recognize childlike fears, feelings, and fantasies without being intimidated by them. It means remaining flexible and open to new experiences despite a Parent whose reply is rigid, overbearing, and authoritative.

Before a health professional can stay in the Adult, it is usually necessary to grapple with an overdeveloped Parent. Our conversations with patients are riveted with "should," "ought," "no," "don't," "never," and "always." Unless you have a strong Adult, it is difficult to resist the temptation to mother, smother, cajole, or control patients.

If you have kept your pencil and paper handy, test yourself on the following patient situation:

> While working on a hematology floor, you enter Jack Stevens's room and find him packing his suitcase. When you ask him what he's doing, he

snaps: "I'm getting the hell out of here! It's been 3 weeks and a million tests, and they still don't know what's wrong!"

How would you respond? Standing there face to face, you would reply, "_____

_____

_____."

If you were in a small group where you *had* to fill in your answer or in which you had to role-play the part of the professional, what thoughts would be racing through your head? Would you be worried that you would not have the "right" reply? Would you be worried that the group might laugh or frown at your answer? If so, you would be feeling a twinge of the NOT OK.

If you left the reply above blank, you may not have wanted proof of your NOT OK in black and white. Please go back and fill in the reply with your own words.

Now look at your response for any intrusion by the Child or Parent. Did you make excuses like "I'm only a practical nurse"? Did you run away from or sidestep the issue? Is your response stiff or stilted? Did you lecture, argue, or try to verbally coerce him into staying?

Here are some responses that have been given to this situation:

"Just a minute, I'll get some help."

"You shouldn't be so upset. We're doing everything we can."

"I know just how you feel."

"You can't do that!"

"If you leave now, you may never know what's wrong. All those tests will be wasted. After all, the doctor wouldn't have ordered all those tests if he didn't feel they were important."

"I'm going for the doctor. We'll see about this!"

"Relax, everything will look better tomorrow."

"I can't stop you, but just remember, you're leaving against medical advice."

Some lecture, some remain silent, but the majority of those responses are peppered with Parent words, phrases, and mannerisms.

Before responding, it is important to recognize that Mr. Stevens is momentarily being controlled by his Child. He is frustrated, frightened, and angry. He wants to run away from the hospital and a dreaded diagnosis. Because he is being "childish," you may automatically slip into the Parent—lecturing, arguing, shaming, threatening. The Parent-Child relationship is scarcely appropriate for parents and their children. When carried over into the professional-patient arena, it can be deadly.

Novels and soap operas feast on the conflict that arises when the patient fails to conform with the doctor's plan. Enter the doctor (Parent Supreme). With righteous indignation, he storms and struts. He lectures, shames, and embarrasses. After his inflamed oration, the patient's eyes are opened. He sees the error of his ways and conforms. The now kindly doctor smiles, and they all live happily ever after.

In real life, however, the outcome is often quite different. The patient may appear to listen and conform, but once out of the doctor's presence, his anger erupts like a volcano. If he is to be treated like a child, he will behave like one. Stubbornly, he may refuse medication, overeat, underexercise, or fail to keep future appointments. He will show the doctor who is in control. Only when he fears death or decay more than the doctor will he humble himself and return. The doctor will shake his head and mutter something about uncooperative patients.

The real-life Jack Stevens did not need false reassurance or thinly veiled threats. Since he was being controlled by his Child, it was essential to first speak to that Child: "It must be very frustrating to go through all those miserable tests and still not know what is happening inside you. You must be frightened," I said. "I can see you're very angry and upset. I would be, too, if I had spent all that time and seemed to be getting nowhere."

These statements were all the permission he needed to vent his anger and frustration. I allowed him to attack the hospital, the doctor, and me without my becoming defensive or retaliating. After his anger dissipated, the fear began to tumble out. He was afraid he was going to die and that we were keeping it from him. Soon his Adult was able to resume control. Together we made a list of all his concerns and questions for the doctor. The misunderstandings were quickly cleared up.

Traces of Parent contamination abound in our health care system. Consider the policies, regulations, and procedures some institutions cling to: keeping vital signs a secret, forcing patients to bathe every morning, making it necessary to sneak children up the back stairs, declining to discuss the cost of care, closing doors when a patient's body is being removed. You can probably add others from your particular health care setting.

My favorite ritual is removing an ambulatory patient from the hospital in a wheelchair. If the patient is unable to make it out of the hospital under his own steam, perhaps he is not ready for discharge. If he is perfectly capable of walking out of the hospital, then this ritual becomes laughable. Sometimes I fantasize wheeling the patient ceremoniously to the curb and dumping him in the gutter. Only a lawyer would claim our responsibility ends there.

Parent-dominated health professionals need to dominate patients. By choosing for patients instead of offering choices, professionals fail to recognize and respect patients as adults and alternately to expect adult behavior from patients. Trapped in a destructive Parent-Child relationship with their patients, they vacillate between duties of nurturing and punishing, depending on whether the patient is being good or naughty. They complain bitterly about patients' draining dependence on them but are intolerant of patients who refuse to surrender their independence. Some of the least helpful professionals are earmarked by their need to always be right or to have the last word. They are overprotective, domineering, rigid, and methodical. They make antiquated customs sacred and threaten anyone who would bring them into question.

As a health professional, you have the right and responsibility to offer patients the benefit of your knowledge and experience—not as a parent figure but as one adult to another. Together as adults you can explore the questions: Who? What? When? Where? Why? How? and How much? The Adult helps the patient to be fully aware of his alternatives, realizing that any final decision belongs to the patient, not to the professional. The Adult can be free to evaluate and alter present customs only when the unquestioned grip of the Parent is broken.

Before you can operate effectively in the Adult, you need to dredge up your Parent and examine its impact on your interpersonal relationships. How do you react to authorities such as teachers, bosses, doctors, or pastors in your own life? Do you tend to become quiet, subdued, obedient, and conforming? Do you find it impossible to talk with them as equals, Adult to Adult? This is part and parcel of the chicken complex: the compulsion to grit your teeth and comply, even when your Adult tells you it is neither useful nor healthy to do so.

To get to the root of the chicken complex, you need to unearth the Child and confront your own NOT OK. When you came into the world, you were naked, small, and helpless. Completely dependent on others to fulfill your needs and desires, you were vulnerable to whatever came your way. You could offer little resistance. As you matured, you became aware of your small stature and powerlessness. You were knee-high without the knowledge, experience, or coordination necessary to fend for yourself, and there was always someone around to remind you of those unhappy facts.

Picture a NOT OK tattooed just above your navel. It becomes a chronic source of embarrassment, and you soon learn that it is customary to conceal it. Over the years, layer by layer, you manage to camouflage your NOT OK. The Parent, Child, and Adult tapes provide partial covering. You gather assorted bits of useful and useless information. You gain experience with all types of people, places, and things. Your coordination improves. (You can even thread a needle!) Shreds of self-confidence accumulate over the sensitive spot. You become taller, stronger, and smarter.

Yet, no matter how convincing your exterior looks to others, you are acutely aware of the NOT OK lurking just below the surface. There is constant fear of indecent exposure. That fear propels you to collect other proof that you are really OK. Look! Credit cards, licenses, awards, references, recommendations, publicity, publications, black belts, merit badges, applause, memberships, diamonds, diplomas, degrees! These decorations fill scrapbooks, walls, and wallets with convincing evidence that you are definitely OK. Perhaps the grandest feather in your cap is your professional qualifications.

Then something happens to tear away at your psychological patchwork. Something goes wrong. You are denied a promotion. Your application is rejected. You fail an exam. You dent a fender. You get a divorce. You lose a patient, forget your lines, burn the dinner, sing off-key. Everyone experiences failure and disappointment.

Loudly, the Child tapes begin to replay familiar strains. Once more, you are engulfed by feelings of loss, failure, rejection, shame, frustrations, or abandonment. Their intensity has not been muted by time. You wither from the blast as devastated as you might have been when you were a defenseless child.

A graphic illustration of the NOT OK in action might be borrowed from one of King Nebuchadnezzar's visions. He had many dreams and visions before he finally went stark raving mad and began grazing with the cattle, but this one seems most apropos. In the vision, he sees a magnificent image with a head of gold, breast and arms of silver, belly and thighs of brass, legs of iron, and feet of clay. While watching the image, he sees a stone hurled that strikes the image on its feet. (Where else?) It topples, is smashed into tiny pieces, and is blown away.

The clay feet are symbolic of the NOT OK. They represent any weak spot in your veneer. You may be a magnificent creature, impressively adorned and confident, until a stone strikes. A stone will bounce off places where you are strongest and best protected, but in the right spot it can wreak havoc, leaving you crippled, demoralized, or demolished.

Unfortunately, some people seem to have an uncanny sense of where you are most vulnerable. Children, lovers, bosses, patients, and parents seem to know what to hurl and when to hurl it. Stones come in many shapes and disguises:

"Why isn't a nice girl like you married?"

"How could anybody be so stupid?"

"My mother never made me sort my socks."

"On you, frizzy hair looks good."

"Just who do you think you are, anyway?"

"Working mothers cause juvenile delinquency."

"Where were you when I needed you?"

"After I gave you the best years of my life. . . ."

"I told you this would happen, didn't I?"

"Ring around the collar."

Some attacks just ruffle your feathers, whereas others strip you down to goose bumps. Damage depends on the severity of the blast and your ability to endure it. It may take a day, a week, a month, or a year to get your feathers smoothed and your facade properly repaired. Protecting the image becomes paramount.

Early in life, some discover that the best defense is a good offense. It is incredible how offensive people can learn to be. Armed with clubs, they set off into the world intent on smashing your toes before you smash theirs. No holds barred. They lop off toes with tongues as sharp as swords—with searing wits, leers, sneers, and slurs. All's fair: shaming, blaming, belittling, ignoring. They slap with stereotype, punch with prejudice, and hit hardest when you're tired, overworked, underpaid, and unappreciated. They will try to expose you for what they are—NOT OK.

If you've tried being offensive, you know it's a full-time job. It's exhausting. In addition, it does little to ease personal pain. No matter how many others you manage to topple, your own NOT OK refuses to be silent. Wearily, you may opt for a different protective mechanism that requires less effort and energy. One of the best is distance. Don't let anyone close enough to hurt you. Don't get involved.

Mugged egos are painful. Just as you learn to avoid physical assault by not walking alone at night in rough neighborhoods, you learn to avoid people, places, and situations in which ego attack is likely. For instance, you hesitate to ask a question that might expose your ignorance, or you keep defective merchandise rather than face a cantankerous clerk.

People in the health professions sometimes protect themselves against ego attack by developing a cool, detached, "professional" exterior. Unfortunately, it is impossible to keep your distance and be therapeutically involved at the same time. To be a helping person, you have to risk closeness. One nurse suggested we should get combat pay because our egos are attacked so often.

The universality of the NOT OK should attenuate its impact. I've got a NOT OK, you've got a NOT OK, everybody's got a NOT OK. That puts us all at an equal disadvantage or an equal advantage, depending on whether you're a pessimist or an optimist. Once you can tolerate the thought of your NOT OK being normal, you are well on your way to disarmament. You will have less need to defend your image or to attack the image of others.

At this point, you are entering Harris's fourth position: I'M OK—YOU'RE OK. This position was not available to us as children. It is an elective position that can only be entered into by the adult. It's the choice you make when you agree within yourself to disarm, to be less offensive and less defensive. Only when you accept yourself can you accept others. Only when you love yourself can you love others.

Although you will never be totally immune to ego attacks, you can practice handling them more efficiently. When stones are hurled, instead of crumbling completely, learn to say, "Ouch! That hurts!" You won't have to waste time and energy seeking revenge, slinking off to lick your wounds, or vowing never to get involved again. You won't have to hide or avoid the people and situations that used to make you so uncomfortable.

Being assertive is only possible when you discover you are more than okay, you're OK! The cure for the chicken complex is learning to accept yourself, respect yourself, love yourself, like yourself. OK?

3

Chicks and roosters

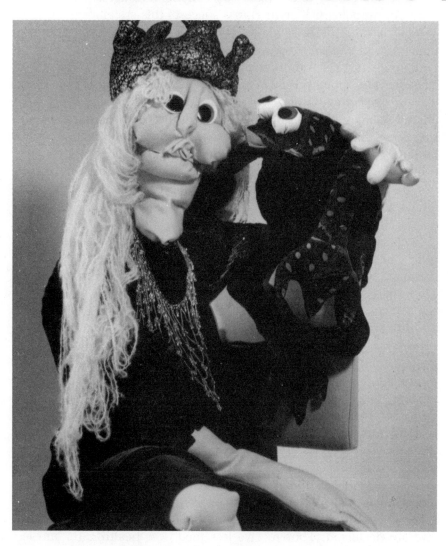

You have to kiss a lot of toads
before you find a prince.

Women have some special problems when learning to be assertive, mainly because we happen to live on a planet where men are dominant and women subordinate. If assertive women are not against God's law, they are certainly against man's.

Male supremacy and female subservience are age-old and world-wide. Anthropologist Marvin Harris suggests this system was invented partially because of the demands of ancient warfare but also, and more important, as a means of preventing overpopulation.

In ancient times warfare required brute force. Since men were usually taller and more muscular, they were trained for hurling and bashing. To make them willing to risk life and limb in battle, the prize offered was sex. Often, only men who had proved themselves as warriors were allowed to marry. A war hero was rewarded with a docile, obedient woman (or docile, obedient women). (Think what a dirty trick it would have been to present him with an assertive woman who would have told him to wash his own clothes because she was running for a seat on the tribal council.)

Warfare helped limit population growth, but it was not sufficient. Other methods had to be devised, and the most effective one seemed to be infanticide—especially female infanticide. The normal birthrate is usually 105 boys to 100 girls. Historians note that less than 100 years ago in parts of northern India the ratio was as high as 233 to 100! In some areas of China, female infanticide reached 80 percent.

In fifteenth-century England, most infant deaths were attributed to suffocation caused by a mother rolling over on her infant. Strangely enough, mothers rolled over on daughters more often than on sons. Infanticide was also common in Germany, Italy, and France, giving new meaning to the phrase: "You've come a long way, baby."

I wish this were all ancient history, but the most recent census statistics compiled by the United Nations suggest that in much of Asia there are only 92 girls to every 100 boys. In China there are 113 boys for every 100 girls. This is especially alarming because we know that in developed countries females are more likely to survive birth and live longer than males. How do they explain the discrepancy? Female infanticide. And, there is overwhelming evidence that girls who do survive are neglected. They receive less food, less health care, and less education than boys.

Today we have relatively safe and certain ways of limiting population growth. We have the knowledge and technology to help preserve natural resources. Brawn is no longer required for modern warfare. A female finger can push a "destruct" button as effectively as a male finger.

Unless suburbs begin marching on each other, it appears that tribal warfare is on the wane. At least in the United States, aggressive men and passive women have outlived their usefulness. Unfortunately, the prehistoric patterning is so strong that we continue to program our children for these archaic functions.

Beginning in the newborn nursery when boys are wrapped in blue and girls in pink, parents and society treat the two sexes differently. The physiological differences between boys and girls pale in importance beside the socialization processes they will undergo in the shaping of the adult man and woman.

Harry Reis, a professor at the University of Rochester, tested 92 preschoolers between the ages of 3 and 5 on their perceptions of masculine and feminine roles. The study consisted of describing a behavior trait aloud to each child. Then the child was asked to point to a silhouette—either an adult male or an adult female—which went with the characteristic.

Traits considered to be masculine included "strong," "adventurous," "self-reliant," "messy," "owns a big store," "brags," and "makes most of the rules."

Children pointed to the feminine silhouette for characteristics like "weak," "talkative," "fussy," "quiet and afraid," "whiny," but "loving" and "well-mannered."

The more things change, the more they stay the same.

Our culture continues to choose to vigorously enhance certain characteristics in one sex while rigorously inhibiting them in the other. Yet inside every man are the seeds of sensitivity, tenderness, vulnerability, and dependence, and inside every woman are the seeds of independence, competitiveness, rationality, and courage. For men or women to have to deny part of what they are or to pretend to be what they are not is unhealthy both physically and emotionally.

Whereas "all men are created equal," women are still struggling with equal rights issues. Even when legal resolution comes, emotional acceptance of equal rights may be light-years away. Because few people are lukewarm on the subjects of equal rights and women's liberation, it may be dangerous to venture into this area so early. Dangerous but essential. Relationships between the sexes must be explored, no matter how briefly, for there to be an understanding of why assertiveness is so difficult for women.

Writing in *The Mismeasure of Woman,* social psychologist Carol Tavris says the fundamental belief in the normalcy of men and the corresponding abnormality of women continues to persist. "In every domain of life, men are considered the normal human being, and women are 'ab-normal,' deficient because they are different from men. It is normal for women to worry about being abnormal, because male behavior, male heroes, male psychology, and even male physiology continue to be the standard of normalcy against which women are measured and found wanting." She goes on to say, "The perception of female otherness occurs in every field, as we are learning from critical observers in science, law, medicine, history, economics, social science, literature, and art."*For a bit of comic relief, look at the following lists she presents†:

What's Wrong with Women	**What's Wrong with Men**
Low self-esteem	Inflated self-esteem
Undervalues her work	Overvalues his work
Gullible	Rigid
Too modest	Too overconfident
No sense of humor	Offensive sense of humor
Selflessness	Selfishness
Works too hard	Doesn't work hard enough
Career line irregular	Career path too narrow
Adult development too erratic	Adult development too conformist
Dependent	Aloof
Too connected, fused with others; weak ego boundary	Too autonomous, isolated, narcissistic
Penis envy	Penis insecurity
Suggestible	Inflexible
Conformist	Unyielding
Too emotional	Too remote, unfeeling
Weak leadership style	Authoritarian leadership style
Unwilling to dominate	Unwilling to negotiate
Stunted moral reasoning	Narrow moral reasoning
Not competitive enough	Not cooperative enough

Tavris says, "Most people will see at once that the negative terms in the righthand column are biased and derogatory, but that is the point.

---

*From Tavris, Carol: *The Mismeasure of Women,* New York, 1992, Simon & Schuster, p. 17. Used with permission.
†Ibid, p. 40.

Why has it been so difficult to notice the same degree of bias and denigration in the lefthand list? The answer is that we are used to seeing women as the problem, to thinking of women as being different 'from men,' and to regarding women's differences from men as deficiencies and weaknesses."*

She is not the only one concerned with how we continue to say women are "sick," while men just have "problems." Psychologist Paula Caplan and sociologist Margrit Eichler were so upset when the *Diagnostic and Statistical Manual of Mental Disorders* decided to include "Self-Defeating Personality Disorder" (SPD), which so blatantly fit society's stereotype of women, they coined another disorder, DDPD or "Delusional Dominating Personality Disorder" (DDPD), which just as blatantly fit men.

To be diagnosed as a self-defeating person, you must meet five of the following criteria†:

1. You choose people and situations that lead to disappointment, failure, or mistreatment.
2. You reject offers of help.
3. You respond to good news or successes with depression, guilt, or actions that produce pain.
4. You provoke others to reject or be angry with you, and then feel hurt, defeated, or humiliated.
5. You turn down opportunities for pleasure.
6. You are able to do well, but you keep sabotaging your own objectives.
7. You reject people who treat you well; for example, you are turned off by considerate sexual partners.
8. You like to play the martyr, sacrificing your own interests for others who do not solicit or need your help.

In an article coauthored with Kaye-Lee Pantomy, Caplan described delusional dominating persons as individuals exhibiting several of the following symptoms‡:

1. They are unable to establish and maintain close relationships.

---

*Ibid, p. 40.

†Modified from American Psychiatric Association: Diagnostic and Statistical Manual of Mental Disorders (ed. 3—rev.), Washington, D.C., 1987, The Association, pp. 373-374.

‡From Pantomy, Kaye-Lee, and Caplan, Paula J.: Delusional dominating personality disorder: a modest proposal for identifying some consequences of rigid masculine socialization, *Canadian Psychology* 32:120-133, 1991. Copyright 1991. Canadian Psychological Association. Reprinted with permission.

2. They are unable to identify and express their feelings and to know how other people feel.
3. They are unable to respond appropriately to the feelings and needs of others.
4. They use power, silence, withdrawal, or avoidance rather than negotiation in coping with conflict.
5. They believe that women are responsible for the bad things that happen to them, while the good things are due to their own abilities or efforts.
6. They need to inflate their importance and achievements (or those of males in general), while needing to deflate the importance of women.
7. They suffer various delusions, such as:
    a. The delusion of personal entitlement to the services of any woman with whom they are associated
    b. The delusion that women like to suffer and to be ordered around
    c. The delusion that physical force is the best method of solving problems
    d. The delusion that sexual and aggressive impulses are uncontrollable in all males
8. They need to affirm their importance by appearing with females who are submissive; conventionally attractive, younger, and shorter; and lower on the socioeconomic scale than they.
9. They have a distorted approach to sexuality, reflected by a pathological need for flattery about their sexual performance and/or the size of their genitals.
10. They tend to feel inordinately threatened by women who fail to disguise their intelligence.

Unfortunately, SPD will be an official "disorder," and DDPD will not.

Basically, women are not programmed to seek success. We are programmed to seek service. When women do act in a manner likely to bring achievement, we are accused of being masculine and, therefore, unhealthy. This is the crux of the problem between women and assertiveness. Assertiveness is thought of as a masculine trait.

Matina Horner's work, which seemed to document women's fear of success in competitive academic or occupational situations, has been reinterpreted by some who suggest her findings may not indicate fear of success as much as fear of sex-role inappropriateness.

Actually, sex-role appropriateness is one issue women in the health professions can handle fairly easily. We have taken all the sustaining, comforting, supporting, nurturing, service-to-others-not-to-self, approved feminine pursuits and made them legitimate careers. But we do have to wrestle with the conflict between having a career or a family, or a combination of the two.

Working women are frequently scapegoats for problems ranging from high rates of divorce to juvenile crime. When we dare step outside rigid sex-approved roles, we are heaped with guilt. Bits of vicious rumor masquerade as scientific fact to frighten us into compliance. Those who are unable to comply because of economic necessity are forced to carry an additional burden.

Separating fact from fantasy about working women is a full-time job. For instance, how many times have you been told that your profession is something "nice to fall back on," with the implication being that for women work is just a passing fancy, something to fill time until the right man or the children come along? It is as though all the training, education, and experience you have had is to be used only in case of emergency.

According to Labor Department statistics, however, the average woman will probably work full-time for 34 years, in addition to marrying and having two children. *Thirty-four years*. That's a long time to be stuck in a low-paying job that offers little in the way of security, fringe benefits, promotion, or advancement. If you are single, widowed, or divorced (as 43 percent of the women in this country are), that number jumps to a whopping 41 years.

Although we know that women are not worthless, we are acutely aware that women are worth less in the economic marketplace. Certainly, one index of the relative value of men and women is income. Today women's median income for full-time work is still only 60 percent of men's income. A professional woman can expect to earn about two thirds of what her male counterpart earns. The gap between men's and women's incomes has not changed despite affirmative action efforts, because 75 percent of all women are in clerical and service jobs that are described as low-paying, low-status, and dead-end.

While women earn the same number of bachelor's degrees and master's degrees as men do, those degrees are concentrated in five fields: home economics, library science, foreign language, health, and education.

For decades the gap between the earnings of women and men remained resistant to change. For years women made 59 cents for every dollar a man made. In the early 1990s, it appeared women were beginning to catch up. We were making closer to 70 cents on the dollar. Then it was pointed out that the reason the gap was narrowing was not that women were making *more* but that men were making *less*.

Profits and pensions have never had a high priority for women. People come first. Putting people first should not be penalized. "We might say that one of the major issues before us as a human community is the question of how to create a way of life that includes serving others without being subservient."* Service without subservience—an idea whose time has come.

Women are people who need people. We value interpersonal relationships above all else and are more likely to consider the needs, opinions, and feelings of others before taking any action. A woman will not think twice about being assertive. She will think 20 times.

Eager to please, a woman is very vulnerable to the You-Can-Be-Perfect-If attack. That's a big IF. For example:

Your husband may say, "You can be a perfect wife IF . . . you sort my socks, balance the budget, always smile, never nag, are superb in both kitchen and bedroom, keep me organized, can BE THERE when I want you, and don't bug me when I'm busy."

Your children may say, "You can be a perfect mother IF . . . you give us freedom, generous allowances, and lots of goodies; keep us entertained; never scream or scold or spank; and can BE THERE when we want you and vanish when we don't."

Your employer may say, "You can be a perfect employee IF . . . you are punctual, hard-working, accept a modest salary, overlook fringe benefits, and can BE THERE at a moment's notice—especially on holidays, weekends, and nights."

Your patient may say, "You can be a perfect therapist IF . . . you are kind and attentive, baby me yet maintain my independence, get me well but don't make me do anything I don't want to do, and, above all, can BE THERE whenever I want or need you."

Be there. Just be there. It seems like a small enough request, until you consider the number of people who demand first place on your list of priorities.

Throughout life, women are expected to organize their lives around the needs of others. The guiding question for a girl is not "What are you going to make out of your life?" but "Who are you going to make?"

As women, we cling to the belief that our ultimate fulfillment lies in

---

*From Miller, Jean Baker: *Toward a New Psychology of Women*, Boston, 1976, Beacon Press, p. 71.

the roles of wife and mother. Perhaps it does. But so does our ultimate frustration.

Studies continue to show that married women have higher rates of mental illness than men, while women who are single, widowed, or divorced have lower rates than men. Evidence suggests that employed, married men are in the best mental health, while unemployed, married women are in the worst. (Employed housewives fall between the two.) Having children in the house seems to contribute to poor mental health.

To stay sane, you need to acknowledge the fact that you cannot be physically and emotionally accessible 24 hours a day without breaking down or wearing out. You also need to recognize that if you spend the bulk of your life "on call," you will not accomplish much of anything else.

Women spend much of life either waiting for someone or waiting on someone. To fill the time you spend waiting meaningfully, you have to make commitments that many women are reluctant to make. They are afraid to get seriously involved in any activity that might keep them from being there immediately when someone they love wants them. So instead of filling time, they opt to kill time with a lethal combination of soap operas, coffee klatsches, shopping, or dusting. When the children enter school, and the number of hours to be killed becomes unbearable, women find that skills to fill time have never been fully developed or have rusted beyond recognition. Many women reach their middle years feeling life has somehow passed them by and moaning, "After I gave you the best years of my life. . . ."

Don't give away the best years of your life. It's okay to share them, but don't give them away. If you have already given away the first 40 years of your life, don't let that stop you from planting and harvesting the back 40. Organizations and self-help groups are available to assist you in entering or reentering the job market.

That reentry process would not be so painful or terrifying if, early in life, women learned to spend some time and thought on their own growth and development. Too often, women's priorities are only reflections of the priorities of others. It is easy to rationalize postponing your own needs and goals until your husband gets a degree . . . until he finds a job . . . until the children are in school . . . until the children finish school.

Having someone to lean on has its drawbacks. Women often learn too late that even within the closest relationships the only person in the world you can rely on completely is yourself. No matter how much you love the man in your life, you are probably going to outlive him by a decade. It pays to be able to balance the checkbook and change a tire or a fuse.

What has been described as "learned helplessness" in women may be endearing in sweet, young things, but it is tiresome and laughable in middle-aged women. As most women mature, they find it more and more difficult to play the "Poor Little Me/Big Strong You" game. Such a game is degrading and nerve-racking.

Women must be allowed to openly appreciate and use their intelligence, ability, and creativity. If these qualities continue to be denied or suppressed, Poor Little Me may feign helplessness but take revenge by continually pointing out the flaws, weaknesses, and shortcomings of Big Strong You.

The passive-aggressive, love-hate relationship between men and women has been called the battle of the sexes. This battle is usually fought with cold-war tactics (sometimes bordering on frigid), but when violence erupts, women are no match for men.

When battered wives were making their first headlines in daily newspapers, I was startled by the bulletin board at the entrance to the medical library. Large, bright letters spelled out "SPOUSE ABUSE," and the table beneath the display was heaped with books and copies of journal articles. My curiosity aroused, I checked the titles of the books. All were about abuse of women. Further intrigued, I took time to sift through the numerous articles. With one small exception, all were about the abuse of women. The only piece I could find to justify the title "Spouse Abuse" was a copy of a brief letter to an editor in which the writer said he had witnessed two cases of husband battering.

The display's title would have been justified if nearly equal numbers of men and women were being battered by their spouses. It might even have been justified if only 90 percent of the victims were women. But when 99.44 percent of the battered are women, "spouse abuse" becomes a euphemism designed to deny man's abuse and misuse of woman.

Used copies of USA Today litter every airport. I never have to buy one. Recently one of their front-page headlines screamed, "Runaway Parents." I read the article and discovered 95 percent of those "parents" were men.

The family is not the only battleground for the war between the sexes. The battle is being fought daily at the local hospital. Between doctors and nurses, the spirit is too often one of conflict and competition instead of cooperation.

When over 80 percent of all physicians are men and 97 percent of all nurses are women, it is easy to see why power struggles between health occupations can quickly disintegrate into power struggles between men and women. In all areas of the health care industry, friction between management and labor boils down to friction between men and women.

While sexual harrassment is illegal, it is still widespread, and it doesn't affect only sweet, young things. It affects powerful women at the top of their professions.

Who can forget Stanford University neurosurgeon Frances Conley? She made national news by resigning her position to protest the impending appointment of a chief of neurosurgery whose choice, she said, would serve "to condone and perpetuate sexism in my work environment." Such a flap ensued that the chief's appointment was withdrawn and she stayed on. According to Conley, "The most difficult aspect of sexism to change is the tendency to stereotype roles according to sex—and to enforce the stereotypes by sexual harrassment."

Fearful of losing their jobs, women often fail to report sexual harrassment. A case made public in January 1993 told of unbelievable harrassment by "the good old boys' network" at the huge Atlanta Veterans Affairs Medical Center that went unchecked for a decade. The top administrators engaged in touching inappropriately, tugging at undergarments, making sexual requests—everything from making comments about one researcher being a member of the "itty bitty titty club" to asking women to help one administrator masturbate so he could get a sample of his sperm for the laboratory!

The VA's inspector general, Stephen A. Trodden, and lawyers who are experts in the field of sexual harrassment have called this case "unrivaled." They said the women were caught in a "Catch-22" situation, because they would have had to have made formal complaints to the very men who were harrassing them. Five officials have been recommended for disciplinary action, and other criminal charges are pending.

Most women find it difficult to be assertive with men. Women in the health professions have to learn to be assertive not only with men, but with powerful medicine men.

Our fragile collective ego not only lets doctors rule the roost in our health care systems, it also allows men to float to the top of professions that are overwhelmingly female.

What kind of men go into nursing? Typically, smart ones: ambitious, intelligent, success-oriented men who want to rise rapidly to the top of some profession. They rarely need assertiveness training. In men assertiveness is expected; aggressiveness is accepted.

When a man begins a job, he looks around and says, "Which way is up?" and begins his climb to the top. When a woman enters a job, she looks down and says, "Look at all this work! I'll never get all this work done!"

Because women value men and men devalue women, women also devalue women. Instead of supporting, cheering, and encouraging each other, we are quick to distrust, belittle, and criticize. Conduct your own poll of colleagues. Casually ask whether they prefer male or female patients. If your results coincide with mine, men will be preferred by a wide margin, and the reasons given will give you firsthand knowledge of some women's prejudices against other women.

Women have had to pretend to be less than adequate so men could feel more adequate. Assertiveness encourages both men and women to meet on common ground: adequacy. Men are OK. Women are OK.

Some suggest nurses continue to play the handmaiden role until physicians are able to accept them as independent, assertive, competent colleagues. If nurses decide to keep playing games, they should be warned that the doctors write the rules and women can never be more than pawns. Women health professionals must take the initiative if we want the right to serve others without being subservient.

As long as I can remember, there has been a push to get more men into nursing. Men were supposed to bring stability, status, and higher salaries. Many intelligent women still feel it is vital to recruit men, not recognizing that this is just a variation on an old theme: What every woman needs most is a man.

Instead of pining away, waiting to be rescued, we had better uncover, develop, and mobilize our own resources if we want to save ourselves and our professions. There are no knights in shining armor, and kissing toads will only lead to warts.

4

Ugly ducklings into swans

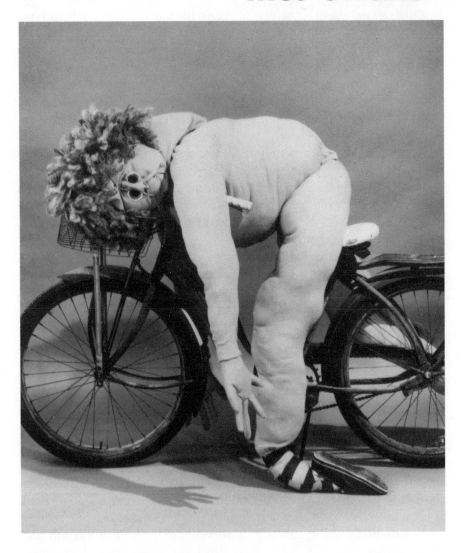

Destiny may shape our ends,
but we shape our middles.

At the end of our graduate program in psychiatric nursing, the instructors invited us over for dinner. That was over 25 years ago, and I can't begin to remember what we ate, but I remember what happened after dinner as vividly as if it were yesterday.

About 20 of us were scattered around the living room when one of the instructors suggested we try something new. We formed a circle and then were told to share one thing we liked about ourselves and one thing we liked about the person on our right.

My stomach flip-flopped, and my brain began whizzing wildly in search of something positive I dared say about myself without sounding pompous or obnoxious. I shot a quick glance at the person on my right and was relieved to find someone I liked very much. My eyes scanned the room, pausing momentarily on each other woman while I fantasized what one thing I would say if she were on my right. For some, a half-dozen good qualities popped into my mind. For others, I was stumped. Suddenly I felt sad that I knew so little about some of my classmates. I regretted the fact that competition between us was often keener than cooperation. I thought it remarkable that I could come so far in life and be more comfortable with criticism than with compliments.

As we began to share, there was some squirming and giggling, but as each person's turn came, there was a breathless silence. All eyes and ears zeroed in on the individual speaker. I wondered if the qualities I had singled out silently would be the ones pronounced aloud.

Those moments were exquisitely painful. I longed to have my turn; yet I was so totally absorbed and fascinated by what was happening inside me and within the group that I savored every moment. The process was as refreshing as a dip in a mountain stream. After the initial shock came intense warmth. As we left that night, I felt we had been given a wonderful farewell gift. It's a gift I would like to pass along to you.

The next time you are with other people, look at them in a different way. Think of what you would say if you had to perform this exercise right then and there. What one thing do you like about yourself that you would be willing to say out loud in front of a group of people? Look at each individual and envision announcing one quality or strength for each of them. Be brave. Actually do this simple exercise at a family dinner, staff meeting, or coffee klatsch. Since most people will be stunned by your suggestion, you will have to take the lead: "One thing I like about myself is _____, and one thing I like about you is _____." You may be surprised at what a difference it can make in your relationships.

To help you get up the nerve to try this out in real life, you may need a boost to your own self-esteem. Take a second look at the list you prepared at the beginning of Chapter 2, when you were asked to list all the things you like about yourself. Look at your list for both quantity and quality. If you are "average," you probably thought of 4 or 5 things you like about yourself. Some women can think of only 1 or 2 things, whereas a rare bird will list 10 or 12. My all-time champion is a nurse who listed 21 items.

More important than quantity, however, is the quality of items and the tone of wording. Many women wriggle out of complimenting themselves by tacking on parenthetical phrases, as in "a good mother (most of the time but not always)" or "personality (half the time)." There is a strong tendency to qualify every item, thus diminishing its importance, as in "usually kind" or "fairly nice." Along with subtle put-downs are blatantly negative expressions. Two favorites in my collection are "fairly rarely depressed" and "not lame or maimed." Many women write backhanded compliments such as "not ugly" and "not stupid." Why is it so hard for a woman to just say "attractive" and "intelligent"?

Incidentally, "intelligent" is conspicuously absent from the lists I have received. Less than 5 percent of respondents list intelligence as one of the things they like about themselves. A television commercial ends with "a mind is a terrible thing to waste." Our minds may not be wasted, but obviously they're often overlooked.

One woman quickly numbered her paper one through five. Next to number one she wrote "honest." The other four numbers she left blank. Apparently, after she had declared herself to be honest she could not "honestly" list anything else she liked about herself.

Another woman also numbered her paper one through five. Next to each number was a squiggly line or doodle as if she had started to write something but had changed her mind. When she reached number five, she wrote, "I'M HAPPY WITH MYSELF!" That's the key: learning to like yourself. If you don't like yourself, you can never master assertiveness.

If you were at a loss for words when you made up your own list, try looking over these words and phrases that have cropped up on lists from other women in the health professions. Circle the ones in the list on p. 36 that apply to you.

Flexible
Loving
Capable
Good health
Well-organized
Efficient
Good influence on my
  children
Woman
Eyes
Honest
Cleanliness
Objectiveness
Ability to get along with
  others and enlist their
  help
Neat
Content
Punctual
Enjoy life
Sincere
Not judgmental
Responsible
Ability to keep a
  confidence
Big boobs
Generous with time or
  money
Kind
Openness
Not afraid to tackle jobs
  that are novel and see
  them through
Initiative
Easy to talk to
I like the way I look
Personality
An easy smile
Reliable
Friendly
Musical talent
Hard worker
Incurable optimist
Good common sense
Weird
Articulate
Good seamstress
Good cook

Slender
Thrifty
Prompt
Do my best
Calm
Intelligent
Ambitious
Good homemaker
Practical
Petite
Confident
Easygoing
Sympathetic
Sensitive
Pleasant
Good speller
Persistent
Craft ability
Loyal
Enthusiastic
Conscientious
Regular exercise
Pride in profession
Natural cheerfulness
Empathy
Great physical
  endurance
Informed
Fair
Curious
Able to delegate
  responsibility
Creative
Eager to learn
Trustworthy
Polite
I'm tall
I can forgive easily and
  not carry a grudge
The age I am in now
Attractive
Emotionally strong
Very perceptive
Capable of talking to
  groups of people
Particular
Soft-spoken
Good problem solver

Adaptive
Meticulous
Strong religious faith
Great body
Candid
Outgoing
Affectionate
Leader
Altruistic
Curious
Tolerant
Versatile
Thorough
Respectful
I accept people as
  they are
Satisfied with life
Tidy
Lost 15 pounds
Ability to concentrate
Know myself
Human
Appreciate nature
Not afraid to talk
  about feelings
Ability to make others
  comfortable in
  tense situations
My hair
Good conversationalist
Good listener
Spontaneous
Mature
Straightforward
Insightful
Poised
Ability to laugh
Resourceful
Experienced
Realistic
Fingernails
Good dancer
Giggly
Sweet
Trusting
Witty
Rich
Alive

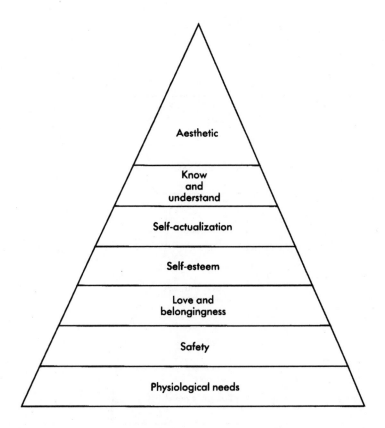

If you are asked to name something you like about yourself now, you should be more than ready. Try sharing this experience with others close to you. We need all the encouragement we can get to look at ourselves and each other in a positive manner.

You are probably familiar with Abraham Maslow's hierarchy of human needs.* It has been reproduced innumerable times. Most often it is diagrammed as a pyramid as shown above.

Every time I see this diagram, I am more convinced it should be drawn like an hourglass instead of a pyramid, with a bottleneck at self-esteem as shown on p. 38.

Ugly duckling or swan, chicken or eagle, NOT OK or OK, the crux is self-esteem. Before you can fly, you have to squeeze through that bot-

---

*Maslow, Abraham H.: *Motivation and Personality,* ed. 3, New York, 1987, Harper & Row, pp. 56-61.

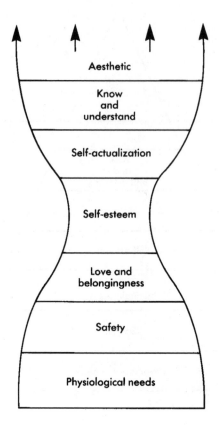

tleneck. The passage is so difficult that few people negotiate it, and fewer women than men make it.

Women, especially those of us in caring professions, tend to be so other-centered that we often lose touch with ourselves. Our self-esteem is an unstable quality that vacillates depending on the mercy of those around us at any given moment. When questioned about who we are, we look to others for our very definition. Each person we ask—parent, pastor, patient, spouse, child, teacher, boss, friend, expert—sees us differently. It is like being trapped in a hall of mirrors. Their images of us conflict. Reality or reflection? There is so much distortion in the eye of the beholder it is difficult to tell.

Paralyzed by fear of what others might think if we stop living up to the image, we retreat from the self-esteem conflict back to the lower levels of safety, love, and belongingness. Unfortunately, there is no way to become self-actualizing while keeping one foot firmly planted in the lower levels.

If you wait for someone else to give you permission to move up in the hierarchy, you will remain forever trapped at the bottom of the hourglass. The only person who can give you permission to move is you. Deciding to move upward is a conscious decision. It involves letting go of some excess baggage—anxieties, fears, defenses, excuses, prejudices, clichés, and rituals. It takes guts to break with tradition and status quo, to step away from others who delight in pointing out your flaws and shortcomings, to give up groveling, wallowing in guilt, or mourning your lack of perfection.

Like Alice stepping through the looking glass into Wonderland, you will find your world altered when you dare confront your reflection. New experiences, feelings, and adventures await you. Entrance into the self-actualization level frees you to become all you can be—not just what you think you should be or, more correctly, what you think others think you should be. At last you are free to explore and learn for the sheer joy of it. You have time and energy to develop aesthetic awareness. The sky's the limit.

A major benefit of working your way above the bottleneck is that it is much harder for people and events to get you down. The passage is so narrow that it is hard to slip back into the NOT OK once you've made the climb. To push you down takes a real catastrophe—not just a snide remark or a bit of tension. You find you are stronger, more comfortable with yourself, and less afraid of involvement, caring, and love. All the things you feared you might lose (safety, love, and belonging) are now open to you in an extraordinarily satisfying way.

People trapped in the bottom of the hourglass will try to discourage you. They will play on your fear and ambivalence. They will try to convince you that everything worthwhile is already there at the lower level. They will tell you that upper-level human needs are reserved for the brilliant, the saintly, the rich, or the gifted. In short, they will say, "You can't get there from here." Don't you believe it. Watch out for those yellow-bellied sapsuckers. Ignore them and keep going.

Luckily, there are some magic words to help you squeak through the self-esteem bottleneck. They were first uttered by Jesse Lair in the book of the same name: "I ain't much baby—but I'm all I've got." Those words may be less poetic than "Shazam!," "Open sesame," or "Bibbity bobbity boo," but they are more functional. At last you have the answer for the person who slaps you with the old who-do-you-think-you-are routine: "I ain't much baby—but I'm all I've got."

Self-esteem should be SELF-esteem. What you think of yourself is much more important than what others think of you. Ugly duckling or swan? You are the only person who can answer. Somewhere along the road to assertiveness lies self-acceptance.

This is it!

This is me!

The only me there'll ever be!

How long has it been since you spent some time with yourself? As women, we funnel most of our time and energy into helping others achieve their goals while we totally neglect our own. We are not even sure we have the right to have goals of our own. We are too busy to indulge our delights and desires. As time goes by, we find it difficult to even remember them. Worst of all, we deny our dreams.

You are a person worth knowing. Find a quiet place, an empty space where you can be alone with yourself. Take time out to rediscover who you are, where you're coming from, and where you would like to go.

Just for fun, try completing the following statements. There are no "wrong" answers if they are *your* answers.

Me!

My favorite color is . . .
My favorite food is . . .
My favorite smell is . . .
My motto is . . .
If I could live anywhere I pleased, I'd be living . . .
My dream job would be . . .
I wish I were bold enough to . . .
Sometimes I wonder if . . .
In 5 years I want . . .
I laugh when . . .
I feel sad when . . .
I get angry when . . .
I am sorry I never . . .
My home is . . .
My favorite people are listed here with one word that best describes each of them:

_____

_____

_____

When I grow up . . .
I love to . . .
My favorite things include . . .
I wish I knew more about . . .
I have never told anyone that . . .
If I were 18 again, I would . . .
I am afraid of . . .
One sure way to lift my spirits is . . .
I am . . .

5

The right wing

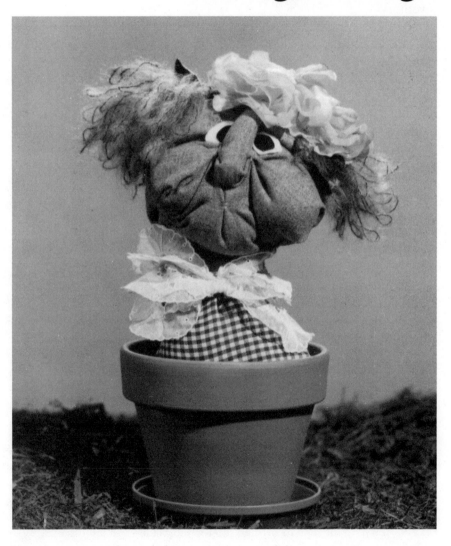

Hold your ground.

T o find out if you can "hold your ground," complete the questionnaire on pp. 65–67. The Nurses Assertiveness Inventory was developed by Larry Michelson, Karen Molcan, and Susan Poorman. The abbreviated questionnaire included in the appendix to this chapter is based on the NAI and is intended for "recreational" purposes. Researchers can contact the authors for the original 84-item inventory.

While the original research subjects were nurses, the questions are relevant to all women health professionals. As you read each question, substitute your profession (such as dietitian, occupational therapist, medical technologist) for the word "nurse." Even if you don't actually complete the questionnaire, you may find that reading through the questions will reveal your assertiveness strengths and areas for improvement.

When the first edition of STAT appeared, "rights" were in their heyday. In fact, the most frequently requested reprint was the list of 10 basic rights for women in the health professions, which is shown in the box below.

However, after years of giving assertiveness training workshops, I tired of talking about rights. While I continued to include them in the handouts, I stopped discussing them. I took them to be obvious and self-explanatory. In short, I took them for granted.

Then something rather dramatic happened. I was giving a workshop for a nationally known medical center. When I checked the handouts, the rights were missing. There was an empty spot on the page where they usually appeared. When I asked the person in charge what

---

Ten basic rights for women in the health professions

1. You have the right to be treated with respect.
2. You have the right to a reasonable work load.
3. You have the right to an equitable wage.
4. You have the right to determine your own priorities.
5. You have the right to ask for what you want.
6. You have the right to refuse without making excuses or feeling guilty.
7. You have the right to make mistakes and be responsible for them.
8. You have the right to give and receive information as a professional.
9. You have the right to act in the best interest of the patient.
10. You have the right to be human.

had happened to them, she became quite flustered. Evidently, the queen of nursing at the institution had read them and found them so threatening, she censored them!

I was more amazed and amused than angry. I felt like the Mennen Skin Bracer commercial where the fellow gets slapped and says, "Thanks, I needed that!"

I don't take the rights for granted anymore. Neither should you. If you don't know your rights, you can't "hold your ground."

The whole issue of rights is the biggest stumbling block to assertiveness. However simplistic it may sound, women are preoccupied with responsibilities, not rights. Devoted to serving others, claiming rights for ourselves seems obscenely selfish. Perhaps the time has come to speak out in favor of a happy medium.

If in reading your rights you feel upset or uncomfortable, you may need some remedial work in the earlier chapters. Resistance to rights is inevitably rooted in the NOT OK. It is one hallmark of those trapped below the self-esteem bottleneck.

The right to be treated with respect

No one has the "right" to degrade, shame, or humiliate another person in public or in private. And no one has the "responsibility" to sit still and take such abuse. It is time to develop a BM Award (Bad Manners, of course) to be given at moments when words are inadequate to express the proper feeling.

Every woman in the health professions should have a pad of BM stickers to slap on the back of a doctor, head nurse, or instructor who has just embarrassed or belittled her in front of patients or colleagues.

What about doctors who scribble illegible orders and then treat the nurses like imbeciles when the nurses have to track them down for clarification? This appears to be an almost universal complaint from nurses in assertiveness training groups. Illegible handwriting is just another example of bad manners. Stick it to them. Unfortunately, this boring behavior can be life-threatening. It should have been nipped in the bud years ago. Physicians who cannot write legibly should be forced to print.

A temper tantrum is a temper tantrum, whether the person involved is a toddler or an eminent brain surgeon. Give the surgeon who throws instruments around the operating room a BM sticker. The rough, the rude, the noisy, the nosey, the bitch, the bully, the gossip, and the grouch—give them all BM stickers.

"A physician was critical of the way I was caring for a patient with a decubitus ulcer. He criticized the way I changed the dressing, the way I positioned the patient, etc. I asked the doctor to demonstrate the way he wanted it done. The doctor quickly found out it was impossible to do it his way. And I found out the doctor had a weak stomach."

While we are at it, perhaps each patient should be given a pad of stickers. I am sure they would love to reward their caregivers and visitors properly.

What's in a name? One nurse wrote: "There have been several times when doctors have either called me by my first name—or nothing—or 'Hey you.' I wish I would have enough 'guts' to call them by their first names."

Her comment reminds me of a lovely, romantic, first-person story published in *Reader's Digest*. It was written by a nurse who had been horribly disfigured in an automobile accident. As a result of the accident she lost her unborn child, and later her husband divorced her. Over the years she had much reconstructive surgery performed by a particular plastic surgeon. Later they worked together professionally. Eventually, he asked her to marry him. Even when he proposed, she couldn't bring herself to use his first name!

Dr. Jonathan Freedman, professor of psychology at Columbia University, conducted a fascinating survey. He polled 2000 doctors, 2000 nurses, and 2000 patients to find out what they thought about each other. One of the most interesting findings was that although nurses found doctors difficult to work with, 85 percent said they respected doctors. Doctors, on the other hand, reported they found nurses easy to work with, but 87 percent said they *did not* respect nurses.

Isn't that what our mothers always told us? Men don't respect women who are easy.

In some instances when women fail to be assertive, they find themselves endangered physically.

"In my last nursing job I was exposed to a fairly high amount of radiation. I was aware of the exposure on accepting the job, but I should have been much more assertive about the amount I would accept and the precautions the hospital took to protect its personnel."

Basically, we are trusting. We expect some authority to be looking out for our well-being. Respect yourself. Look out for yourself.

Ignorance is not bliss. It's dangerous. Be knowledgeable first. Don't rely on others' authority. Get facts straight.

Respect yourself enough to speak up. By brooding in silence, we make mountains out of molehills.

"As part of an orientation plan in a smaller hospital, I was told by the director of patient services to work a few times on each shift on both the medical and surgical floors. While I was setting up the schedule with one of the head nurses, she commented: 'I don't know why you are being oriented to this floor. We have more help than we need now.' Apparently there was a lack of communication somewhere, but I continued to have an 'unwanted and outsider' feeling. I wish I could have had a proper yet respectful reply."

The assertive response is simply to put into words what you are thinking and feeling. For instance: "There seems to be some lack of communication here. The director just wants me to get acquainted with both the medical and surgical floors. I feel rather awkward and unwanted." The head nurse was probably unaware of the impact of her words. Getting your feelings out in the open saves a lot of misery and misunderstanding. You will most likely get an apology.

"Whenever I start work in a new hospital, I'm always a little quiet. People have mistaken this for lack of intelligence or being stuck-up—of which neither is true. Consequently, I get stuck with all the work, all the shifts, and all the extra duty. Being a newlywed, my husband didn't appreciate it, and he was the one who finally forced me to stand up to my superior for equal time off with my co-workers. It is difficult for me to speak with superiors—nursing directors, doctors, and others."

Pick up on the word "superiors." If you feel "inferior" to others, it is impossible to assert yourself.

Overemphasis on educational background is a real sore spot among women in the health professions. Intellectually, we know that there are some grossly incompetent people with PhDs and some incredibly competent people who never finished high school. Emotionally, however, many of us are intimidated by degrees or lack of them. Let's begin to give each other credit, not only for educational background or rank or salary, but for ability to perform well on the job, integrity, tact, skill, dedication, and compassion. The most important things in life aren't reflected in college degrees.

The right to a reasonable work load

Nurses have reported being called at 2 or 3 AM and being asked to come in to work. One exhausted nurse took her phone off the hook. At 6 AM someone pounded on her front door. When she looked out, she saw the police. Her first thought was that a family member had been killed in an automobile accident.

When she opened the door, the officer said, "Call the hospital. They have been trying to get you for hours. Your phone must be out of order."

The staffing office had sent the police to see if she would come in to work on her day off!

All of us will pitch in and work extra during times of emergency, but some hospitals are in a perpetual staffing crisis. This kind of management, or rather lack of management, destroys human resources.

When Cynthia Knox (not her real name) first took the clinical nurse specialist position at a metropolitan children's hospital, she was excited by the challenges and possibilities. The job description read like a dream. Who could have known the dream would soon prove to be a nightmare?

Her primary responsibilities were to teach, counsel, and guide the staff, along with the children and their parents. She was to develop research proposals, as well as aid in ongoing research. She was to help design the ideal children's unit, working closely with the architects, since construction was scheduled to begin within the year.

The new unit was desperately needed. Hers was always over-crowded. Too many children, too few nurses. Soon she found herself working nights, weekends, and occasionally double shifts. Having worked as a missionary in an underdeveloped country, she was not averse to hard work. She was highly skilled, efficient, and compassionate. She poured body and soul into work. Her time and energy were sapped just by the physical care of the children. There was little left over for counseling, teaching, planning, or research.

Exhausted, she went to the administration, which sympathized and promised to ease the situation. No help materialized. In desperation, she threatened to resign. The administration countered with: "It is bad enough now. Think what will happen if you leave, too. Who will care for the children?" That kept her in line for a few extra months.

After almost 2 years of back-breaking, heartbreaking work, she resigned. Broken in spirit, humiliated, and guilt-ridden, she found refuge in a small, private school where she teaches pediatric nursing.

The Cynthia Knox situation is not uncommon. A major complaint of women in the health professions is overwork. We leap into our careers brimming with enthusiasm and burn out before the year is up.

Some of us flee from our professions physically. I found one social worker selling clothing at a local department store. She could no longer cope with the stupendous responsibility and the skimpy support. The harsh realities of the health care system force many of us to hide out in schools and universities where we can busy ourselves with the intellectual pursuit of the ideal. Housewives who have been trained in the health professions are reluctant to return to their careers, even when able, because the rewards are so few and the sacrifices so great.

Some of us flee from our professions emotionally. We all know professional zombies who burned out years ago but continue to work in the health professions. You can recognize them by their dull eyes, mechanized routines, lack of involvement, and refusal to question the status quo. Their bodies are warm, but their hearts are cold, and their minds are frozen.

The system may be at fault for much of the overwork, but part of the problem we bring on ourselves. Inability to delegate responsibility ties many women up in knots.

"When working in a small general hospital, I found it easier to do things myself than to make sure the staff got them done and done right."

Or:

"When I was a head nurse, I found it very difficult to say no to requests for special hours, and I would work shifts that were short of help. I ended up with bad effects on my physical and mental health. I do not like to offend anybody."

Another problem contributing to unreasonable work loads is the inability to reprimand or dismiss workers who are not doing their share.

"It is difficult for me to reprimand a worker in my charge whom I think is not doing her work satisfactorily. This is something I really need help with now in my position as a nursing supervisor. I have difficulty asserting myself as an authority when criticism is involved."

This nurse echoes the dilemma of the nurse who does not like to offend anybody. We have all covered for fellow workers. We can do our work and theirs too for a short time. If the problem is chronic, however, anger and resentment are inevitable. Morale slips.

How do we reward good workers? We give them more work. How do we reward incompetent workers? We give them less work.

Three faculty members were complaining about "their" secretary. While she did good work for the department head, she did lousy work for them. For example, when she typed their class materials, she made so many errors they had decided it was just easier to do it themselves.

They had rewarded her for incompetence. They did her work for her. Instead, they should have insisted she do the work over and over until she got it right. It wasn't that she *could not* do the work properly, she *would not*. If she continued to sabotage their work, she should have been terminated.

Here's the sad tale of another secretary:

> "Our secretary is outspoken, overpowering, dictating, and rude—but does an excellent job. I tried counseling her myself, but it didn't work. She has a lot of personal problems, and losing this job would make matters worse. What can I do?"

My first question would be: "Does an excellent job" of what? How can a person who is "overpowering, dictating, and rude" be an asset? Often the secretary is the primary link between the institution and the public. A secretary like this can do a lot of damage to an organization. At best, she is a horrendous public relations problem.

The wording suggests the secretary has some skills and the manager sees potential. To salvage her might mean something as simple as sending her to training classes in customer relations. Or she might be switched to a more suitable job, somewhere in the bowels of the hospital, where she can deal with things instead of people.

When the manager worries about the secretary's "personal problems" and fears "losing this job would make matters worse," she is making the classic mistake of letting personal circumstances interfere with professional decisions. She is trying to be both boss and therapist—a combination that rarely works.

She needs to be firm about job performance expectations. As for therapy, she needs to refer her secretary to professional help.

When it comes to reprimanding a worker or firing her, the guiding question has to be: **Is what I am doing or about to do in the best interest of the patient?** This question may help break the hold of the "Mother Hen Superior" complex. We cannot take care of everyone.

Our primary responsibility is to care for patients. Anything or anyone interfering with that responsibility has to go.

Here is another situation to consider:

> "My problem is my nursing supervisor. I am a shy, happy-go-lucky person but efficient and dependable. For this reason, I am literally pushed around from one department to another, with no consideration for my convenience, fears, or discomfort at having to work in unfamiliar departments. The supervisor's only concern is filling the vacancy so she will look good. She cares nothing about the cost to me.
>
> When I once mentioned I thought I should be compensated for this, I was given a strong put-down. I work part-time for a large clinic as a relief nurse. From my viewpoint, I am cheap labor (I get no benefits). How I would love to go higher up and speak my mind, but I am not assertive or articulate enough to do this."

The first sentence is the tip-off. Instead of blaming the supervisor or the system, there must come an honest owning up: "My problem is me." As any assertive woman will tell you, *once* is not enough. Get one-paragraph references about your work from each department. Approach your supervisor again. If she fails to respond, go to her supervisor. If they do not improve your situation or compensate you adequately, quit. Or settle down to work in a less than perfect situation knowing that you have done your best.

The sad part about many inequitable situations is that if you quit, they will just bring in another nurse and treat her the same way. When she refuses to be exploited, another nurse will come along. The clinic cannot lose. They have an overready supply of cheap labor. The patients are the losers. What are we going to do about it?

The right to an equitable wage

Determining an "equitable" wage is tough. According to the dictionary, it means coming up with a wage that is "just, impartial, and fair."

Unfortunately, there seems to be very little rhyme or reason to the way wages are set on this planet. Only a few years ago the Department of Labor's *Dictionary of Occupational Titles,* the United State's most widely used tool for setting wages, ranked the jobs of nurse and parking lot attendant as equally complex.

Nurses always seemed to get the short end of the stick. They could justifiably whine about their salaries. For example, a nurse in Chicago who just completed a PhD degree was feeling a little low. It seemed the pop truck drivers had been out on strike, making it impossible to return pop bottles to the grocery stores. As part of the settlement, the drivers received a salary that was higher than hers!

When asked, "Yes, but would you want to be a pop truck driver?" she wondered why no one ever asked, "Yes, but would you want to be a nurse?"

Female physicians who read *Megatrends for Women* may begin to ask themselves that very question. Authors Patricia Aburdene and John Naisbitt site Bureau of Labor statistics to suggest that "in 1991 women nurses earned more money than nonentrepreneurial female physicians."* (By the way, 63 percent of women doctors are "nonentrepreneurial," meaning they are on salary.)

"Yes, doctor, but would you want to be a nurse?"

In 1988 *Working Woman* placed nursing on its list of worst jobs. By 1991 nursing was on its list of best jobs. Salaries improved dramatically, but that improvement seemed to go unnoticed by the majority of nurses. Whenever I ask a nurse how much she *should* make, the answer is always the same: "More!"

"More" is not an acceptable answer. As major health care reform looms on the horizon, nurses may have to scramble to keep the economic gains they have made from eroding.

All of the women in the health care professions—doctors, nurses, physical therapists, dietitians, social workers, lab technicians—need to work assertively to establish wages that are "just, impartial, and fair." Given the Department of Labor's track record, we should not leave this task to them.

The right to determine your own priorities

Whether on the job or in your personal life, you have the right to decide what your priorities are. You have the right to choose the ways in which you spend your time and energy. If you waver, a host of other people will be happy to make the choices for you.

"Because I take a commitment seriously, I was careful to attend all meetings of our United Way last summer. I completed my responsibility, and at that point I was pressured to become the secretary, because to them I seemed very interested because of my regular attendance at meetings. I

---

*From Aburdene, Patricia, and Naisbitt, John: *Megatrends for Women,* (New York, 1992, Villard Books, p. 72.)

was successfully assertive and refused the position, because I feel my place is at home during the hours right after school. It was difficult for me to be assertive, but I felt satisfaction afterward."

As women, we are receptive and responsive to the needs and desires of those around us. This is both an asset and a liability. After finally getting her sixth child off to school, one woman was delighted to learn that she had been accepted into graduate school. A week later she sadly reported that her husband had vetoed her returning to school because it might interfere with *his* plans. As women, we should be entitled to some dreams and plans of our own. If you really want to return to school or to work, your needs and desires should have equal consideration.

"When the director of nursing found out I was taking a medication course on my days off, she said, 'That will do you no good here!' I simply replied, 'I may not always be here.'"

It's difficult to give patients top priority with all the minor interruptions we have to deal with daily.

"A patient was crying. When I asked her what the problem was, she said nothing. Again I questioned her, and she pushed me away. I was then called to the phone and detained for 20 minutes. I wasn't able to follow through on her problem. I wish I had had someone else take the phone call and had tried to determine her problem with another approach."

Electing to stay with a patient who needs you may well mean refusing or delaying other tasks. Women in the health professions are still trying to be in two (or more) places at once. We tend to give in and do things to please parent figures—completing paperwork, assisting physicians, and so on—rather than helping patients.

"Five years ago, I discovered a lump in my breast and consulted an excellent surgeon. He and I agreed it should be biopsied, although he said he was 90 percent sure it was benign. I told him at the time I would sign a consent form for the biopsy only. If it were malignant, I would make a decision only when I knew what the alternatives were.
   I think he felt that I was questioning his ability. I wasn't. I felt that I needed more time to prepare myself and my family for the more serious and debilitating surgical procedure. After some convincing arguing, he agreed to do the biopsy only and let me make the decisions that I felt were

mine to make. Fortunately, the biopsy was benign. Despite the disagreement, we are friendly when we meet."

It is important to have some control over your job, your time, your body, your life. Be able to say to yourself: "This is right for me. This is right for me now." Life is ever changing. Be brave enough to change with it.

The right to ask for what you want

Although there can be no guarantee that you will get what you want, you certainly have the right to ask for it. Whether you crave a night on the town, help with a new procedure, some time alone, or a specific patient assignment, wishes must be put into words before they can come true. Women often keep silent, thinking others should sense what they want or need. It is disappointing how few mind readers there are in the world.

Suffering in silence can be hazardous to your health.

"About 20 people were crammed into a small conference room when one woman began to smoke. The smoke was particularly irritating to me. I wish I would have asked the woman to stop—I didn't."

Why do nonsmokers still find it so difficult to ask smokers to refrain from smoking? The evidence that cigarette smoke is harmful to nonsmokers is very convincing. Even armed with this knowledge, often we are still reluctant to infringe on another's rights. Before you get angry enough to douse someone with a bucket of water, simply express the fact that smoke really bothers you. Most smokers will be polite enough to stop, if they are asked openly and politely. If they don't, present them with one of your BM stickers.

During job interviews, you may be asked to temporarily accept an assignment other than the one you have requested. One nurse who wanted to work in a coronary care unit was "temporarily" shunted to an orthopedic unit. Six months later she was still in orthopedics and angry to learn that two new nurses had been placed in the coronary care unit during that time. The moral is to keep your requests visible. Out of sight, out of mind. Make sure you check in with the nursing director every few weeks to see if there is an opening on your desired unit.

After working for several years, Peggy decided to return to graduate school. She knew she could no longer work full-time and had been keeping her eyes open for a good part-time job. She found the ideal job—one that would not only mesh with her schedule but meant fascinating work with top-notch professionals.

Since there were several qualified applicants, Peggy waited anxiously for the decision. Finally, she called the supervisor, who apologized for the delay and told her they had narrowed the field to two candidates. Peggy was one of them!

Peggy told the supervisor how thrilled she was to be one of the final candidates. Then Peggy asked if there was anything she could do to help with the decision-making process. She offered to come in for a second interview and concluded the conversation saying, "I *really* want this job. I know I can exceed your expectations."

Peggy's husband overheard the conversation and was startled by his wife's assertive behavior. He did not think that it was appropriate for her to speak so boldly, and he thought that she had blown her chance.

Guess who got the job. Peggy.

Here is another good example of asking for what you want:

"Our recently handicapped child attends a therapy session established to last 1 hour. However, the therapist was always late and frequently dismissed the child early. Questioning these shortened sessions, I was told that there was no financial loss, since insurance pays the bill. I reminded the individual that indirectly I was paying and said that, to be truthful, she wasn't giving of her skill in a complete and honest manner. Because I respected her abilities and did not display hostility, we are both comfortable in meeting now, and our child is getting proper therapy."

Don't pout or fume silently. Speak up quickly, calmly, honestly. It's your right.

The right to refuse without making excuses or feeling guilty

Refusing to collect for a charity when an anonymous telephone solicitor asks you to is a relatively easy task. It is difficult to refuse a request from a friend or co-worker and even more difficult to refuse a request from a supervisor.

One nurse shared her exasperation at always being called in on her day off. We did a role-play of the situation, and the next time her head nurse phoned, this is what happened:

"I wondered if you could come in and work on Friday. It looks like we'll be short-handed again."

"This is the third time this month I have been called to come in on my day off. I will not be able to work this Friday."

"Oh . . . do you have special plans?"

"No, but I need a break from work. I plan to take my day off."

"But who will I get to help out if you won't come in to work?"

"I don't know. I am sure it is difficult for you."

"Yes, it is! We are always short of help. I know we need to hire another nurse, but it just isn't in the budget. Are you sure you can't come in on Friday?"

"I'm sure."

"Who can I get to cover?"

"I don't know."

"Oh, well . . . I can probably find somebody. I'll see you later."

The nurse felt very good after this exchange. No lying, no lame excuses, no ulcer attack, no migraine headache. Most women are more than willing to help out in a pinch, but many report being constantly taken advantage of and then being made to feel guilty and selfish when they begin to refuse.

Giving questionable dosages of medication is a frequent problem brought out in assertiveness training groups.

"I refused to give a medication ordered, because I felt the dosage was excessive. This put me in line for great verbal abuse by the doctor. Although somewhat intimidated, I said if he insisted on that dosage, then he would have to administer it himself, since I refused. He finally wrote an order for a more reasonable dosage. Although I had visions of a lot of repercussions, it actually made for more mutual respect. I have never forgotten that situation."

Here is a similar situation that went unresolved:

"A general practitioner who limited practice to psychiatry habitually prescribed large dosages of medications for his patients. On one occasion, he ordered medications that I knew should not be given together. I questioned whether he wanted them both given, and he answered yes. Instead of administering the medication, I wish I had refused to do so. This doctor would never admit his own fallibility. If questioned, he would never change his mind. However, a day or two later, he would change his orders."

Many women health professionals have real problems with authority figures. Even in situations where our own education, experience, and judgment run contrary to what we see the authority doing or saying, we are still reluctant to openly oppose or question what is happening. In any of these situations, ask yourself, "**Is what I am doing or about to**

do in the best interest of the patient?" That should give you the needed courage to lay your ego on the line.

> A clinical psychologist was asked to participate in a panel discussion on women and mental health. The selection committee had suddenly realized they had an all-male panel and that, given the topic, it would probably be wise to include a woman. With only 2 days to prepare and a 3-hour drive to consider, the psychologist declined. Earlier in her career, she said, she would have jumped at the chance, because she would have been so flattered to have been invited. Now she found she was comfortable enough with her ability and worth to decline the invitation.

Last but not least, you also have the right to refuse to be assertive. When you choose not to assert yourself, you need offer no excuses or explanations. You have the right to refuse.

The right to make mistakes and be responsible for them

Women health professionals seem almost terrified of making mistakes. No amount of education or experience seems to override the NOT OK fear of being wrong. This unreasonable fear prevents us from questioning authorities, speaking up, or stepping in on behalf of the patient.

Penalties for minor errors on the job can be so ego shattering that many women are afraid to admit mistakes. Fully conscious that human lives are involved, we agree that there is no room for error. But everyone makes mistakes—the most skillful surgeon and the least skillful nurse's aide. Never being wrong should not be more important than doing right. Maintaining an infallible image is never in the patient's best interest.

An occupational therapist came upon a man who had had a heart attack. Others were standing around. No one seemed to know what to do. She froze. Even though she had some long-ago training, she couldn't bring herself to act. The ambulance arrived just moments later, but the man died. The woman felt extremely guilty. After kicking herself around for quite a while, she finally resolved to do something positive. She enrolled in a CPR course taught by the Red Cross and has gone on to become one of their instructors.

Another woman told of assisting at the scene of an automobile accident near her home.

> "I felt the ambulance volunteers (untrained) positioned the man poorly to transport him to the hospital. I questioned them. He died. I felt that perhaps if I had been more assertive—could he have lived?"

There is no way to answer her question. She, like many other women health professionals, hesitated and later was haunted by the question of what might have been.

Besides professional examples, many come from personal lives.

"When my daughter was having trouble in first grade, I felt she should be retained and suggested this in a conference with both her teacher and principal. She was not retained. Many times since that decision, I have regretted my submissive inaction."

"Submissive inaction" is a very descriptive phrase for what happens to many of us. Decisions affecting you and your family belong in your hands. It is wise to seek expert advice, but the final decision should be yours. Right or wrong, it will be easier to live with your decision than with someone else's.

Finding yourself in a bad job can be just as painful as finding yourself in a bad marriage. It is difficult to admit you have made a poor choice or a poor decision. Instead of resigning yourself to living with your mistake, face up to the situation, take responsibility for the error, and then work on a solution, or a "divorce."

I am not sure if it is loyalty or masochism that binds so many women to joyless, thankless jobs. The health professions have a way of making mincemeat out of bodies, minds, and spirits. Our dying words are, "If I don't do it, who will?" Perhaps if there were no one willing to sacrifice herself in vain, the job situations would be altered, and patient care would improve.

If you find yourself caught in a job that is asking either too much or too little of you, break away. There are bound to be work situations better suited to your needs, talents, abilities, and interests. I just hope they are within the health professions.

We can all help create a climate in which mistakes can be admitted, knowing that colleagues will be quick to help and slow to condemn. Belittling or shaming will only drive mistakes underground, making corrections almost impossible.

The right to give and receive information as a professional

We have come a long way from the days when nurses were not even allowed to disclose a patient's temperature or blood pressure, but we still have a long way to go. Being professional cannot be a sometime thing. Nurses often complain that their "professional" status depends on the time of day. During the day, doctors seem to have little regard for the nurse's opinion. At about suppertime, the nurse suddenly becomes much more knowledgeable and astute in her judgment. After 10 PM, she becomes near genius in her ability to diagnose and treat patients.

Remember that you have the right to approach any other person in the health professions as one professional to another. This can be especially important when telephoning.

"We recently received a patient from a hospital on the fourth day after a leg amputation. She didn't have a dressing on her stump. Her past history showed frequent postoperative infections. I felt she should have a dressing and called the surgeon's office. I never got beyond the receptionist. Within the next 48 hours, the patient had two involuntary stools, contaminating her stitches. Three calls later, we still didn't have an order for a dressing, but we put one on anyway. The surgical site became infected, and, would you believe it, it took us a week to get an antibiotic order! The patient had to return to the hospital for treatment of her infected wound. I feel if I had been more assertive and had demanded to talk to the doctor, maybe some of this could have been prevented."

Not being able to get beyond the receptionist can be a real problem. Here is how one woman solved it:

A social worker was caring for her terminally ill father at home. She found it almost impossible to get through to the doctor on the telephone. His receptionist insisted that she explain the problem to her, and she would pass it along to the doctor. Several messages seemed to have been mislaid or erroneously reported, so the social worker began insisting on speaking to the doctor directly.

She listened patiently to each excuse the receptionist gave but firmly refused to speak to anyone but the doctor. When the receptionist finally ran out of excuses, the social worker said: "I telephoned the doctor twice yesterday, and he never returned my call. I plan to call every 15 minutes until I am able to speak to the doctor directly." Ten minutes later, the doctor phoned and apologized for the delay and the misunderstandings.

Persistence, perseverance, and a bit of imagination paid off.

What do you do when a co-worker is giving misinformation to patients? Correct them in private if possible. The most important consideration, however, must be the patient's welfare. If the incorrect information is potentially harmful, you have the right and responsibility to intervene on the spot.

"A very confident nonprofessional explained her 'knowledge' of someone's illness. I knew that all her facts weren't correct, but I remained silent."

"I help with the Senior Center Blood Pressure program. I know I should be more firm in advising these people to see a doctor, take their medication, stay on their special diets, and so forth. I feel I'm too wishy-washy with them. I don't want to treat them like children, so I do not like to scold. When I finish, I feel as if I didn't get through to them."

How do you give information without talking down to patients, scolding, or threatening them? The answer is to talk with them as one adult to another. Share what you know in an open, forthright manner. "If you take your medication, this is what you can expect. If you don't take your medication, then this is what you can expect." If the patient refuses to act on the information, that is his or her right.

Often a little problem solving goes a long way in these situations. You may need to call and make the doctor's appointment right then and there, being sure a ride will be available when the time comes. You may need to find a place to keep a medication in plain view, so they won't forget to take it, or to enlist the help of Meals on Wheels to ensure a proper diet.

The right to act in the best interest of the patient

In the case of no other right will you be hit as frequently with the old who-do-you-think-you-are dodge. Women in the health professions are too easily intimidated. You have lived a long time, had professional training and perhaps years of professional experience. When it comes time to stand up to a doctor, administrator, or family member, don't be so quick to back down.

You do have the right to act in the best interest of the patient. Here are five situations that illustrate the importance of this right. Consider each. How might you have reacted under the same circumstances?

Situation A

"At 3 AM a patient 3 months' pregnant called her doctor to report cramping and spotting. He told her to go to work in the morning as usual. At 8 AM the patient came to work. She called me. She was upset, frightened, and felt something was wrong, but she was afraid to 'bother' her doctor, since he didn't seem concerned and was impatient with her. I then spoke to her doctor. He didn't want to be bothered—said it probably wasn't anything and not to take her too seriously.

I was furious about this lack of concern! I felt this patient should be examined and, if it indeed wasn't serious, at least be reassured. So, feeling this way, I consulted the obstetrician who was on call that day and explained her symptoms. He agreed that she needed attention and told me to send her to the hospital immediately, where he performed a dilation and curettage at 8:45 AM.

I realize that I could have gotten myself into a lot of trouble, because I went over Doctor 1's head to Doctor 2. However, I believe the patient comes first. In this case, I was successfully assertive."

Situation B

"I work with retarded residents who in recent months have been transferred from crib-type beds to low beds without side rails as part of a normalization program. I spoke to my supervisor about getting side rails for those who have frequent seizures and have been known to fall out of bed, but I received no satisfaction. Finally, after one of the girls fell and sustained a laceration requiring sutures, I spoke with my supervisor again and then communicated with her supervisor. Side rails have now been placed on the bed of that particular resident. I wish I had been more assertive sooner."

Situation C

"I was successfully assertive in a professional situation when it was very unusual for a nurse to question a doctor's orders. Following a myocardial infarction, a patient with a very low blood pressure was receiving fluids with aramine added intravenously. The amount of aramine added was so low that we were giving the man too much fluid. I questioned Dr. C about this when he reordered the same strength. He thought and then doubled the amount of aramine. The next time I saw Dr. C, he came up and told me I was very right to question him about his order."

Situation D

"On coming on duty one morning as charge nurse, I immediately checked on a patient who was reported as 'not so good' by the night shift. After checking his vital signs and level of consciousness, I knew that he should be moved to the Intensive care unit to receive the constant attention he needed. His personal physician disagreed. When his consulting physician arrived shortly afterward, I again stated my views. The doctor took one look at the patient and ordered him moved to the ICU as fast as possible. The patient remained in the ICU for more than a week."

Situation E

"As a young nurse I was working part-time in the operating room. A woman with severe viral pneumonia receiving continuous oxygen was brought down for a tracheotomy. The floor nurse left her in the hallway, taking the portable oxygen tank with her, after being assured the patient would be in the OR in less than 5 minutes. Her color was bad, and she had to sit up to breathe. I tried to talk the OR nurses into connecting our oxygen tank, but they didn't want to contaminate it. I brought it out from the storeroom but couldn't find tubing and mask and was told to take it back. The patient finally got into the OR 35 minutes later and died before the tracheotomy could be done."

I am sure this nurse has wished a thousand times that she had gotten oxygen for that woman, even if it meant running naked through the halls screaming like a banshee. But it is too late. If you really care about patients, forget your pride. Don't be afraid to question what you see happening to them. Hold your ground until you get results.

When resources are limited, acting in the best interest of the patient may require a tough decision involving *which* patient should be served. Here is a stunning example:

"It was a holiday. Everything that could go wrong on the unit was going wrong. We have an eight-bed ICU, and in 2 hours seven patients turned over.

Everyone had ended up in the room of a catastrophic patient. Wild, heroic measures were being taken. Everyone was absorbed by the high drama. The team was about to institute a last-ditch intervention that would not reverse the patient's condition but would sustain the patient in this miserable state indefinitely.

The head nurse said quietly, 'Ladies and gentlemen, we have viable patients across the hall who are dying.'

There was a moment of silence. Treatment was suspended. We resumed caring for the other patients, who had momentarily been forgotten in the crisis."

The right to be human

A mature woman with two young children was in her third year of medical school. When the children became ill, she found it necessary to drop one of her courses. Even though she was an excellent student both clinically and academically, the assistant dean whom she had to consult quipped: "You will never make a good doctor. Your family is too important to you." This unkind, inane remark bothered the student so much that she sought professional counseling. The counselor quickly discerned that it was not the student but the dean who needed professional help.

As important and vital as our careers may be, they should not be expected or allowed to obliterate all other facets of our lives. You have the right to sample and enjoy things other than work. To understand patients, it is helpful to have a variety of life experiences.

You are human. Not a saint. Not a martyr. Not a genius. Not a superwoman. Not a super anything. Just a human being.

Many women share times when they were less than perfect in dealing with other people. Even as they recall the events, it is clear that they still harbor guilt resulting from incidents that took place years ago.

> "When the doctors sort of said my dad was terminally ill, and Dad felt it, I wish I could have accepted it and talked with him more, instead of trying to mask the truth and be lighthearted."

You cannot be the perfect professional all the time. You can never be professional with members of your own family. You are human. You must grieve and cope and learn. These are your rights, too.

Because you are human, you will get tired, sloppy, impatient, crabby, giddy, greedy, excited, and scared. You will make mistakes. You will not always care deeply about every patient or person in your life. You will not always have power to make the lame walk, the mute talk, or the blind see. Life and death are not under your control. This is not failure. It is just being human.

A public health nurse tells of a patient who simply stopped walking five years ago, although he had no physical impairment. Complications resulting from his inactivity now make it impossible for him to walk. The nurse feels frustrated and guilty because she cannot help this man. She feels responsible for his problems, even though she has only cared for him a short time. It is important to sort out people who want to be salvaged from those who do not. We squander a lot of time and energy trying to save people who do not choose to be saved.

The plight of humans trying to be superhumans may be reflected in this saying posted in an outpatient clinic struggling to keep chronic schizophrenics out of institutions and in the community:

> "We, the willing, led by the unknowing, are doing the impossible for the ungrateful; we have done so much for so long with so little, we are now qualified to do anything with nothing."

The issue of rights can easily become lopsided. Rights need to be tempered with responsibilities. Responsibilities need to be rewarded with rights. We already have a Bill of Rights. What we need is a Bill of Responsibilities:

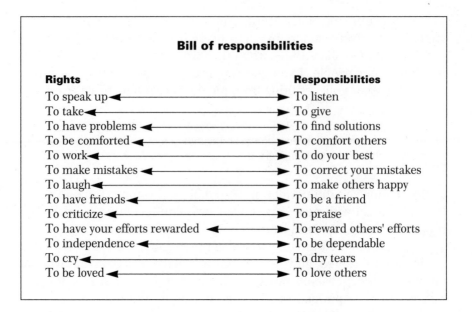

Take time to add your own ideas for "Rights-Responsibilities." It really is a two-way street. The assertive person knows that abusing either one is destructive to the whole person.

Appendix

Nurses Assertiveness Inventory

The following questionnaire is designed to provide information about the manner in which you express yourself. Please answer each question by circling the appropriate number from 1 to 5 (1— Never/Rarely, 2—Seldom, 3—Sometimes, 4—Usually, and 5— Always or Almost Always) on your answer sheet. Your answers should reflect how you generally express yourself in the situation.

	Never/ Rarely	Seldom	Sometimes	Usually	Always or Almost Always
1. If you were preparing medication and your co-workers (also nurses) were making too much noise and interrupting your concentration, would you ask them to stop?	1	2	3	4	5
2. If you are angry at a patient, can you tell him?	1	2	3	4	5
3. If you were in a nurse's meeting (small group) and the nurse supervisor made a statement you thought to be unfair, would you disagree?	1	2	3	4	5
4. If a physician you respect expresses opinions with which you strongly disagree, would you state your opposing opinions?	1	2	3	4	5
5. If a co-worker (nurse) makes what you believe to be an unreasonable request, are you able to refuse?	1	2	3	4	5
6. Do you have difficulty complimenting co-workers (nurse) on a job well done?	1	2	3	4	5
7. If things are just not going right on the unit, would you express your dissatisfaction to the nurse supervisor?	1	2	3	4	5

Reprinted from *Behavioral Research Therapy* 24:1, Michelson, Larry, Molcan, Karen, and Poorman, Susan, "Nurses Assertiveness Inventory," pp. 77-81, © 1986 with permission from Pergamon Press Ltd., Headington Hill Hall, Oxford OX3 OBW, UK.

Continued.

Nurses Assertiveness Inventory—cont'd

	Never/ Rarely	Seldom	Sometimes	Usually	Always or Almost Always
8. If a nurse supervisor were annoying you with numerous requests, would you hide your feelings rather than express your annoyance?	1	2	3	4	5
9. A patient is being unfair; would you say something to him?	1	2	3	4	5
10. Are you able to defend your personal rights with physicians?	1	2	3	4	5
11. Are you able to defend your personal rights with co-workers (nurse)?	1	2	3	4	5
12. Do you have difficulty complimenting a nurse supervisor on a job well done?	1	2	3	4	5
13. Do you have difficulty complimenting a physician on a case well managed?	1	2	3	4	5
14. A nurse supervisor is being unfair; would you say something to her?	1	2	3	4	5
15. Do you find yourself keeping your opinions to yourself rather than expressing them to a physician?	1	2	3	4	5
16. If a person unfamiliar to you walked into the nurse's station wearing a lab coat and requested a patient's chart, would you hand him the chart?	1	2	3	4	5
17. If a physician hurts your feelings, can you express your feelings to the physician?	1	2	3	4	5
18. If a nurse supervisor hurts your feelings, can you express your feelings to her?	1	2	3	4	5
19. If a physician criticizes you and you become angry, can you express your feelings?	1	2	3	4	5

20. Is it a problem for you to maintain a conversation with a physician?   1   2   3   4   5

21. If a co-worker (nurse) criticizes you and you become angry, can you express your feelings?   1   2   3   4   5

22. Is it a problem for you to initiate a conversation with a new employee (nurse)?   1   2   3   4   5

23. Do you speak up when a physician orders a medication that you believe is inappropriate?   1   2   3   4   5

24. If a patient criticizes you and you become angry, can you express your feelings?   1   2   3   4   5

25. Do you find it difficult to express your feelings to a physician who has just treated you in an inferior manner?   1   2   3   4   5

26. Do you find it difficult to ask for a favor from a co-worker (nurse)?   1   2   3   4   5

27. Do you find it difficult terminating a conversation with a patient?   1   2   3   4   5

28. Do you find it difficult terminating a conversation with a co-worker (nurse)?   1   2   3   4   5

29. Do you become embarrassed when a physician tells you that you look nice?   1   2   3   4   5

30. You are standing in line in the cafeteria and a nurse's aide steps in front of you; will you defend your personal rights?   1   2   3   4   5

31. Do you find it difficult terminating a conversation with a physician?   1   2   3   4   5

32. Do you find it difficult terminating a conversation with a nurse supervisor?   1   2   3   4   5

Scoring the Nurses Assertiveness Inventory

For half the questions, the higher the number you circled, the higher your assertiveness score. For example, if you circled a 1, 2, 3, 4, or 5, that number is your score. This applies to questions 1, 2, 3, 4, 5, 7, 9, 10, 11, 14, 17, 18, 19, 21, 23, 24, and 30.

For the other half of the questions, the point value is reversed. For example, if you circled Number 1 (Never/Rarely), you would give yourself 5 points; Number 2 (Seldom) is worth 4 points; Number 3 (Sometimes) is still worth 3 points; Number 4 (Usually) is worth 2 points; and Number 5 (Always or Almost Always) is worth 1 point. This reverse scoring applies to questions 6, 8, 12, 13, 15, 16, 20, 22, 25, 26, 27, 28, 29, 31, and 32.

There are 160 possible points. If you scored in the lower third, you should run, not walk, to the nearest assertiveness training class. You are in desperate need of help! If you scored in the middle third, you have probably already taken an assertiveness class. Keep up the good work, you are going to be just fine! If you scored in the upper third, you should not be reading an assertiveness book, you should be writing one!

6

Learning to fly

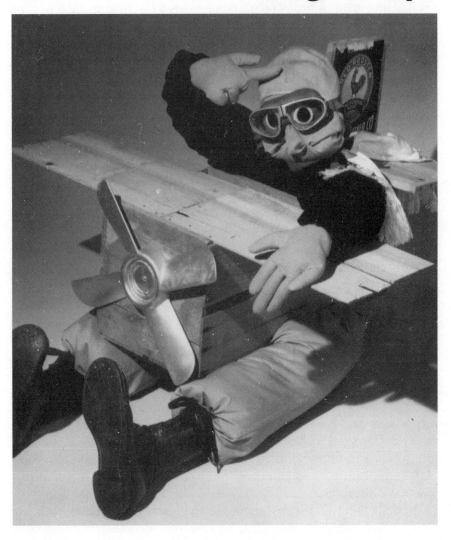

*Flying's easy—
it's getting off the ground that's hard.*

Flying is easy. It's getting off the ground that's hard.

Begin by reading everything you can get your hands on. Articles on assertiveness training appear in newspapers, magazines, and professional journals. Self-help books have sprung up like mushrooms on your bookstore shelves. To help you tell the palatable from the poisonous, an annotated bibliography is provided at the end of this book.

Reading about other people's problems is a fascinating pastime, and you can gather lots of valuable information on the dos and don'ts of assertiveness. After you consume a few paperbacks, you will notice how repetitious some of the principles are. The case studies vary, but the formulas for assertive behavior are simple and almost standardized. Examine the problems and situations described for tips on how you can help yourself. Some techniques will appeal to you more than others. After studying assertiveness, do something about it.

That transition between thinking and doing is a difficult one. To help you get off the ground, I strongly recommend participation in an assertiveness training group. Groups also have sprung up like mushrooms, and there is bound to be one near you. You can watch the newspaper, or you can be assertive and call the YWCA, your local mental health association or community college, or any psychiatrist or social worker. Tell them you are interested in attending an assertiveness training class or workshop.

Participating in an assertiveness training group will put you in touch with other people who are working on finding the happy medium between being passive or aggressive. It is nice to know you are not alone. A group can give you the support and encouragement you will need to get over your fear of flying.

Often one of the first exercises is to have each member introduce herself to the rest of the group. Immediately, you will see that there are some people who are more bold, confident, and positive than others. Not only do you get a chance to observe others for assertive characteristics, but they get a chance to observe you and give you feedback. The group acts as a mirror to help you see yourself as others see you. They can often pick up clues and cues from your manner and behavior that you would overlook.

Initially, you will work on some fictional exercises, such as having to interrupt someone, sharing differing opinions without being passive or aggressive, exchanging merchandise, or asking for a raise. Later you will work on real-life situations suggested by group members themselves. This gives assertiveness an immediacy and a reality that reading cannot match.

Most of us have experienced moments we would like to relive. Group role-play gives you another chance to work through sticky situations. It gives you a chance to say the things you wish you had said, to do the things you wish you had done. This practice prepares you for handling future situations more effectively. The group is also a great place to share "the thrill of victory and the agony of defeat."

Books and groups are important, but they are merely a means to an end. They are not meant to be an end in themselves. Some people have difficulty with this distinction.

Louise is a groupie. She has been a member of one kind of self-help group or another for the past 5 years. She says she gets nervous if she isn't attending sessions of some kind every week. She shuttles from one group to another in hopes of finding some simple magic that will catapult her out of her colorless life.

During the group session, Louise seems genuinely interested in improving herself. When the group session is over, however, she slips back into her rut, complaining that she just can't seem to get started.

Don't be like Louise. Get started. Recognize that assertiveness training is not magic. It is not a cure-all. It takes work, not wishes, to pull it out of theoretical limbo and into everyday living.

Start. Start small.

A colleague thanked me for telling her about a new assertiveness training book I had been reading. She had just finished reading it and exclaimed ecstatically, "After 42 years I finally know how to handle my mother!" Of course, "handling" her mother backfired, and she returned quite sober and dismayed. She was ready to give up assertiveness after one skirmish. Skirmish? It was more like a war.

Let me amend my advice. Start. Start small. Start with strangers.

In relationships as intricate and as intense as mother-daughter, being suddenly assertive can be disastrous. The other person sees an abrupt change as threatening and will probably see your action as aggressive instead of assertive. Becoming assertive in these relationships requires a good deal of thought and planning. Role-playing in your group can help you avoid major catastrophes. Before leaping off a cliff and flapping your arms wildly, take time to gain some experience and confidence.

For your first assertive adventure, pick a person with whom you have no emotional investment and whose approval or disapproval should not matter to you. Pick a small situation that has been bothering you, perhaps one involving telephone solicitors, door-to-door salesmen, waitresses, receptionists, or car mechanics.

A good example might be that of the ward clerk at a sprawling state institution who was often sent to the administration building to make copies of certain files. One woman, whose desk was only a few feet from the copying machine, never failed to interrupt her and ask permission to "just run a few copies."

The interruption was so consistent it really began to bother the ward clerk. She felt herself getting more and more angry about it. She brought the situation to the group and received several suggestions. The group role-played some of the alternatives, which ranged from confronting the woman with her behavior to just saying calmly: "Yes, I would mind. I will be done in a few minutes."

The ward clerk decided to confront the woman. The next time the interruption occurred, the clerk said pleasantly: "I know this sounds funny, but you interrupted me Tuesday, Wednesday, and twice yesterday while I was using the copier. I'm beginning to feel a little paranoid."

The woman laughed and apologized. She has not interrupted the clerk again, and they smile and speak when passing.

> "One doctor always did procedures at the change of shift. When I asked him to come at a different time, he refused, saying his time was important and that he couldn't please all the people.
>
> Using reverse psychology, I began paging the doctor every day at 3 PM to let him know we were ready to assist him. We weren't ready, of course, but he never showed up when paged, so it worked out perfectly."

With assertiveness, nothing succeeds like success. Nothing will give you more courage to be assertive than handling minor daily incidents. Being bold, confident, and positive really pays off.

> "A few weeks ago I received a call from the administrator of a nursing home where I had worked for almost 3 years before I left 6 months ago. Their new dietitian had suddenly become ill, and they needed an immediate replacement.
>
> I surprised the administrator (and myself) when I asked for a certain salary. He was silent for a moment and then said he would call me back the next day.
>
> I got the salary I asked for! Had I not asked, I would have been hired at the former salary, and I would never have known it was possible to get more just by being assertive and asking!"

Another asset pays off even more—persistence. You can get more mileage out of persistence than out of almost any other assertive technique.

As a security measure during the Persian Gulf War, airports suspended curbside check-in for luggage. It was a minor inconvenience. It meant I had to wrestle my bags up to the counter. When I told the agent I would check two bags and carry on the two small ones, she informed me I was only allowed a total of three bags. She said she would have to charge me $30 for the extra one.

I was very surprised. No one had informed me of that before. I asked her to show me where that was written.

She flatly stated that had always been their policy. They just hadn't been enforcing it. I repeated, "Show me where that's written." She began scanning the fine print on the ticket jacket and was frustrated when she couldn't find anything.

She called the supervisor over, who affirmed the three-bag policy. I asked her to show me where that was written, insisting that if I had been aware of the rules, I would have packed differently or chosen another airline.

The supervisor began examining the fine print, muttering over and over that it was a long-standing policy. I told her I flew 100,000 miles a year and if that was the rule I needed to know it, so, "Show me where that's written."

After looking over various documents, they still couldn't find the written policy. They finally gave up and checked my luggage at no extra charge.

On the surface it seems simple enough, but getting women in the health professions to be persistent is incredibly difficult. We bend over backward to see the other person's point of view. We hate to offend anyone. We pride ourselves on being fair, flexible, and open-minded. Someone quipped that we try to be so open-minded our brains fall out.

Getting women to speak up is easier than getting them to stand behind what they say. At the first sign of conflict (an icy stare, a questioning look, a put-down, a refusal), women beat a hasty retreat. Before you retreat, repeat what you said. Once is not enough. Twice may not be enough. Repeat your case over and over again in a calm, even voice. Do not become angry or argumentative.

"I discovered that a co-worker with approximately the same status but fewer years of service and experience earns 88 cents an hour more than I do. I approached the personnel director. I thought I was assertive as I stated my case and asked for job comparison—capabilities, productivity, etc. I was promised something would be done. Nothing came of this. I've also done nothing more."

This example illustrates the importance of setting time limits. Granted, the personnel director might not be able to correct the situation on the spot, but he or she needs to know you expect action—soon! As you are concluding your session, say, "I will check back with you on Thursday morning."

On Thursday morning if there is no resolution, say, "I will check back with you on Tuesday afternoon." This confident approach will make it impossible for the administrator to conveniently forget your plight.

Persist. Persist cheerfully. The director will soon tire of your appearances and resolve the issue.

> Two weeks before the dietitians' conference, Elizabeth shipped six boxes of brochures and other materials to the hotel where she would be staying. When she arrived and asked for her boxes, her heart sank when she was told they had no boxes for her.
>
> Elizabeth insisted the boxes must be there and urged the assistant manager to check again. Panic mounted as she waited for his return. Hundreds of participants would converge on the conference, and she would have nothing to give them.
>
> The assistant manager returned and stated again there were no boxes for Elizabeth.
>
> "If the boxes were here, where would they be?" Elizabeth asked.
>
> "They would be in the storeroom. But I tell you your boxes are not there."
>
> "Take me to the storeroom," she replied.
>
> "I checked for the boxes myself. Yours are not there."
>
> "Take me to the storeroom," she persisted.
>
> Exasperated, the assistant manager complied.
>
> The minute the door opened, Elizabeth spotted her boxes. It was an honest mistake. The recycled boxes had been commandeered from a manufacturing company and were covered with deceptive advertising. The assistant manager had simply glanced at the boxes and concluded they did not belong to Elizabeth. He hadn't bothered to check the shipping labels.

In many instances it pays to be a woman of few words. State what you want or what is bothering you in as few words as possible. The fewer words you use, the more difficult it is to argue with you. If you remain steadfast and single-minded, you will not be lured off into tangents or sidetracked by smooth talkers who wish to cloud the issue.

> "Our unit needs another nurse."
>
> "Do you know what would happen if every unit in the hospital requested one more nurse?"

"No, I do not. I just know that our unit needs another nurse to give safe patient care."

Once you decide on the course of action that is in the best interest of the patient, stand up for your decision. If you persevere, you may be surprised at how quickly others will retreat or at least withdraw to reconsider the situation. Being flexible is fine, but many situations in life require backbone.

"While working in a small hospital in eastern Oregon, I received a phone call at home from the Director of Nurses asking me to accompany a patient with a severed spinal cord and a tracheostomy on an ambulance trip to the university medical center about 100 miles away. I had been his floor nurse on the 11 PM to 7 AM shift the past few days, and the patient had indicated he had a lot of confidence in my nursing care. His construction company would pay $100 to the nurse who went on the ambulance trip. Another nurse had indicated that she wanted to go in my place.

I had worked all night, and the phone had awakened me. My initial reaction was that I felt too tired and sleepy to go on the trip, which was to start right then. After I hung up the phone and felt more awake, I knew I wanted to go and called the director back. She said I would have to call the nurse who was taking my place. This nurse insisted on going herself because, she said, she needed the money. I gave in and let her go in my place. I later found out she was not very interested in what kind of patient care she gave.

I felt I had let the patient down by not going after he had requested me to be the one to go. The patient was very apprehensive about his tracheostomy and depressed because he was a paraplegic from a construction job injury he had just received. I have always regretted my not being more assertive with her."

In this situation, the second nurse outpersisted the first nurse. The money and the fact that the first nurse had momentarily refused to make the trip are side issues. The crux of the matter, and the point that cannot be argued, is the fact that the patient requested her to go with him.

To handle this in a more assertive manner, she should listen politely to every excuse or argument the second nurse gives and then calmly and steadfastly repeat: "But the patient requested me, and I intend to go with him."

When the second nurse says she needs the money, the first nurse should reply, "I am sorry you are disappointed, but the patient requested me, and I intend to go with him." When the second nurse reminds her that she initially turned down his request, she should say: "That is true. But the patient requested me, and I intend to go with him."

After three or four exchanges, the second nurse will see that the first nurse has no intention of backing down and will drop the matter. She may be angry and disappointed, but the patient will be appreciative and relieved. When it comes to offending someone to defend the patient, there really is no choice. If you let the patient and yourself down, you will be haunted by another I-wish-I-had-it-to-do-all-over-again situation.

Here is an excellent example of assertive persistence in action:

> "Last summer I visited my son and his wife and joined them at their church picnic. Lots of people and happy children.
>
> I noticed one child who was continually scratching. His mother told him not to scratch: 'It'll only make it worse!' I went over and looked. I even asked him to raise his T-shirt. His body was covered with large hives. I told the mother the child should be taken to a doctor. She replied, 'Oh, he probably got into some nettles. They'll go away.'
>
> But I didn't like the look on the child's face—it was apprehensive. I followed the child's movements for about 5 minutes and saw his frantic efforts to scratch and yet try to resist that urge. The hives got bigger and spread over his arms and onto his face.
>
> I approached the mother again. She really wasn't that alarmed and said she would apply cold compresses. I told her I was a nurse and I really thought the child needed medical attention. She informed me she would go ahead with the cold compresses. I cornered the minister and told him the child might be in danger and why. He was more persuasive with the mother than I, and she did take her son to the hospital emergency room.
>
> A week later, I got a very nice note thanking me for urging medical attention for the child. She informed me that they had almost lost him because of the severity of the reaction."

This woman had enough guts to speak up and to keep speaking up until she got results. After the initial rebuff by the mother, she didn't just shrug her shoulders and say, "Oh well, I tried, didn't I?"

Follow this woman's example. Don't make a half-hearted attempt to be assertive and then be disappointed when it doesn't quite work. Throw body, soul, and ego into what you are doing. If you sit in a corner and wait until you get enough confidence to be assertive, you will be covered with cobwebs. Confidence comes *after* you dare to assert yourself. The more you assert yourself, the more confident you will become. The more confident you become, the easier it is to be assertive.

"I had a supervisor who completely misunderstood a letter I had written him. He replied with a two-page, typewritten statement of why I was not worthy to exist, let alone continue in my job.

The next day I went to his home, determined to stay until I was able to talk with him face to face. We had an open, honest confrontation.

Even though he had a wide reputation for being 'difficult,' we became best friends. For the rest of his life, I never made a major decision without consulting him, and he became very protective of my welfare."

When learning to be assertive, the use of "I" is imperative. How else can you articulate true feelings, needs, and expectations in an unmistakable manner?

I feel . . .

I expect . . .

I want . . .

I choose . . .

I decide . . .

I plan . . .

I believe . . .

I am (angry, confused, delighted, disappointed) . . .

"I-messages" tend to be less threatening and more effective in keeping communication open than "you-messages." For example, consider the difference between each of the following pairs:

"I get so angry when promises are broken!"
"You make me so mad! You never keep a promise!"

"I appreciate your opinion, but I believe this is best for me."
"You ought to mind your own business."

"I expect you to pick up your dirty clothes."
"You are such a slob! Look at this mess."

Pretend you have received an unfair grade and have decided to talk with your instructor about it. As you enter his office, which words would invite explanation without threatening or blaming?

"You made a mistake in my grade."

"Why did I get a C?"

"I don't understand my grade."

The first response is an accusation that automatically prompts the instructor to defend his position or deny the problem exists even before he investigates it. The second response is also less than optimum, because "whys" are always threatening and usually irrelevant. In this case, the third response would be best.

The following situation revolves around just such an unfair grade:

> After years as a homemaker, Martha returned to college. She thrived on hard work and was making excellent grades. In her anthropology class, however, she was aware of a "personality clash" with the young, male instructor. For some reason, he simply didn't like her no matter how hard she tried to please him.
>
> On all of her exams, projects, and written assignments she had received A's and B's. You can imagine her surprise and disappointment when she received a C for the course.
>
> Unfortunately, Martha did nothing about her grade. Six years later, the incident was still bothering her enough that she asked her assertiveness training group to help work out step-by-step actions that could have helped her prevent this nagging conflict.

The group devised the following six steps as the best course of action for anyone caught in a similar situation:

1. Don't take the grade personally (at least initially). Assume the best, not the worst.
2. Gather documentation: tests, projects, papers.
3. Make an appointment. Approach the instructor with "I am puzzled about my grade." Make no lengthy arguments or explanations.
4. Wait calmly. Give him time to check his grade book. Remember, it may be an honest mistake. Even if he did it maliciously, he has a face-saving way out by blaming the error on a secretary or a computer. The "why" is not important. Your only concern is acquiring the correct grade.
5. After presenting your documentation, if he still refuses to alter the grade and you are unsatisfied with his reasoning, say, "I disagree with your assessment of my performance. I will speak to the division chairman."
6. Follow through. Stay centered on the task and avoid any temptation to lapse into personality conflict.

It may take 5 minutes to remedy the situation. It may take 5 weeks. Any effort is a small price to pay to avoid 6 years of brooding.

Exploring all the "should haves" is useful if what you learn can be applied to new situations. It is not useful to torment yourself with "I wish I would have said . . . ," "I *should* have . . . ," or "Why didn't I . . . ?"

Once the grade becomes ancient history, as it has for Martha, there is only one thing left to do: GET OVER IT. That's another motto suitable for framing.

The courage or timidity with which you handle strangers is some indication of how difficult it will be to assert yourself with the important people in your life. Before you move assertiveness into close relationships, imagine the most awful thing that could happen. The extremes usually involve getting a divorce or getting fired. Conjuring up dire consequences this way makes most women realize how unrealistic and exaggerated their fears are. They discover they have been passive to protect their pride and to keep their "nice woman" and "good mother" images from being tarnished.

Once you decide to be assertive with your family and friends, start slowly and start small. Your new behavior is bound to be questioned or attacked. If you are unsure of yourself, you may suffer a setback. Even if you make a crash landing the first time or two, don't give up.

Naturally, there is some risk in altering your behavior. Change is always threatening, but it can also be invigorating. Here is a beautiful example of assertiveness within close personal relationships:

> "My sister-in-law, who is 45 years old and mentally handicapped, has been living with us 6 months out of the year since her mother died 3 years ago. She promptly began changing our daily lives (we have five children) through temper tantrums, demands, and general uncooperativeness (wouldn't allow me to wash her hair or clothes, wet the bed on purpose, and so forth).
>
> She stated, 'You're not my sister, and I don't have to listen to you.' I was admonished by her brother and sister to be glad my children were normal and to accept Mandy as she was.
>
> After 8 weeks of great tension, I decided that this unhappy situation must change for my own sanity and the happiness of our children, who saw all of Mandy's whims being met while they were required to adhere to good manners, sharing, and working together.
>
> I asserted myself by explaining to Mandy and the relatives that this was our home, too, and we were entitled to enjoy it, and that meant Mandy must adjust. We praised her for any good she did and took away privileges, such as her daily bottle of pop (before, she freely demanded up to five bottles a day at one point) or TV watching or dessert, for misdemeanors. I insisted she participate in our area center for the handicapped against much family anger.
>
> Mandy has adjusted quite well, and the daily problems we do have I feel I can cope with because I am in control again. Life here is much better now since I asserted myself after realizing 'This is my home.' Mandy has lived

up to our increased expectations of her in many ways, and we are back to loving each other."

A lot of perseverance went into turning this destructive situation around. It has the happy ending that many women report when they finally break out of the passive-aggressive-guilt cycle: "We are back to loving each other."

Once you learn to fly, there is no telling how far you can go. Like Nancy Talley, for example, who became the first nurse in Florida to hang up a shingle and go into private practice. When she consulted attorneys in 1972, she was told there was no precedent for nurses in private practice. The issue went all the way to the state attorney general, who determined that if there was no precedent, there was also nothing to prohibit it.

Nancy opened her practice and became an activist working for legislation that would clearly define a role for advanced nursing. In 1974 the "Advanced Registered Nurse Practitioner" category was established.

By 1976 Nancy had launched her own company, Professional Counseling and Consultation Service, in Tampa. Over the past 17 years her company has grown and prospered. She laughs when she recalls how she initially called herself a "counselor" because "psychotherapist" seemed so presumptuous. Today she has a thriving practice and is very comfortable with the title psychotherapist.

Do not limit your options because there are no precedents. Be a pioneer. Fly!

7

How to tell a turkey to stuff it

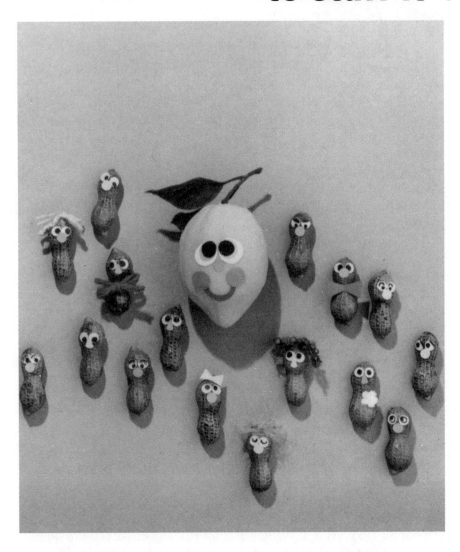

You don't have to be nuts to work here.

What's the most difficult word in the English language to pronounce? For many, it's "no."

Recently, whole books have been devoted to teaching men and women how to say no. That seemingly simple goal has also been the focus of countless assertiveness training groups.

A popular criticism of assertiveness training is that it just gives an excuse to people who are already bullies to go ahead and take advantage of other people. On the contrary, the goal of assertiveness training is not to help you take advantage of other people, but to stop other people from taking advantage of you. And the quickest way to stop people from taking advantage of you is to say no.

The necessarily negative flavor of all this has turned off some women. They sense a rather belligerent and uncaring aura around assertiveness. It is true that many women, while learning to be assertive, go through a negative phase much like the one toddlers experience. That little word "no" has incredible force. Even when you were only 2 feet tall, you could bring things to a grinding halt by saying no. For the adult woman, it is like recapturing some long-forgotten power.

Like using an atrophied muscle, the more you exercise your prerogative to say no, the easier it becomes. First you find you can refuse requests on the telephone and later face to face. You begin by saying no to strangers and progress to friends and family. Ultimately, you are able to hold your own with assorted authorities, such as bosses, teachers, doctors, and even the clergy. Hallelujah!

But the purpose of assertiveness training is not to turn you into a no-it-all. Anyone who doesn't progress beyond the negative phase has a case of arrested development. The beauty of assertiveness is that it frees you to say yes. Yes to all the people, places, and things you really want to get involved with.

It takes some time and effort to understand assertiveness. Throughout the years, we have been conditioned to label behavior as either passive or aggressive. We are now realizing that sandwiched between those two extremes is a third area: assertive behavior.

There is a lot of talk about the fine line between being assertive and being aggressive. Women are petrified that they will cross this line without even knowing it. Whereas it may be uncomfortable to be passive, it is abominable to be aggressive. If this is worrying you, take heart. The line between assertiveness and aggressiveness is not as fine or as fragile as you may think.

Consult any dictionary, and you will find some interesting words and phrases used to define *assertive* and *aggressive*. *Assertive* is defined with words like "bold," "confident," and "positive." *Aggressive* is defined with words like "hostile," "injurious," "violating," and "destructive." It is difficult to believe there is much danger of confusing the two. The dictionary does list *aggressive* as a synonym for *assertive*, but that is merely cause for semantic stumbling, not for stumbling in real life.

> "I was waiting for morning report when the night nurse came in to tell the group something that was not on the taped report. Everyone, including me, was busy chatting. She spoke my name loudly and said, 'Shut up! I'm trying to tell you something!'
>
> I immediately shut up, and so did everyone else. She was very assertive, but I was not. I did not know what to say."

The night nurse in this situation was not assertive. She was aggressive. By the time you finish this chapter, you will have a good idea of what to say to a person who humiliates you like this in front of others.

In today's jargon, passive behavior has been labeled "nonassertive," that is, behavior that is not bold, not confident, and not positive. I prefer to use "passive" instead of "nonassertive." The dictionary defines *passive* as lethargic, inert, submissive, exhibiting no gain or control, and receiving or enduring without resistance. That seems much more descriptive and accurate when talking about women in the health professions. We have been lethargic, inert, and submissive. We have no control over the health care system, and we have endured much abuse and misuse without resistance.

No dictionary will give you the following definition for *turkey,* but for the purpose of this book, a "turkey" will be defined as anyone who wants to take advantage of you: anyone who wants to gobble up your time, energy, talent, money, patience, goodwill, humor, or self-respect. Rediscovering the word "no" is an excellent beginning in learning to deal with the turkeys in your life.

For example, the telephone rings, and you are asked to collect for the Annual Athlete's Foot Fund. Assuming that no one close to you is suffering from terminal athlete's foot and that you really have no interest in their annual drive, how will you respond? You have three basic options: passive, aggressive, or assertive.

The passive response (lethargic, inert, submissive) is to listen to the entire spiel, offer weak excuses (each of which is expertly dismissed by the solicitor), and finally give in and agree to march for athlete's foot, kicking yourself every step of the way.

The aggressive response (hostile, injurious, destructive) might be to curse, belittle the cause, slam the receiver down abruptly, or rip the phone off the wall.

The assertive response is to say, "No" or "No, thank you." Offer no excuses, but boldly, confidently, and positively decline. Being assertive, you will already have offered your time, talent, and financial backing to organizations that really do interest you. This type of positive action on your part will go a long way toward easing any guilt feelings you may have about not being able to save the whole world.

There is certainly nothing wrong in agreeing to collect for a charity, *unless* you feel angry with yourself for doing so. After hanging up the phone, many women are furious with themselves for not being able to refuse anyone anything.

The passive woman usually finds her life cluttered with odds and ends that no one else wants to do. She has never learned to value herself, much less her time. Although she doesn't actively seek additional chores, she has never learned how to refuse effectively. Her silence is taken as consent.

She believes in giving until it hurts. Even when it hurts, she continues to give until the pain is excruciating. Then comes the straw that breaks her back. Some minor request or inconvenience suddenly sets her off like a skyrocket. There is an emotional holocaust, with shaming, blaming, screaming, and crying. Afterward, she usually feels intense guilt. Ashamed and remorseful, she quietly slips back into the passive routine. Her life might be diagrammed like this:

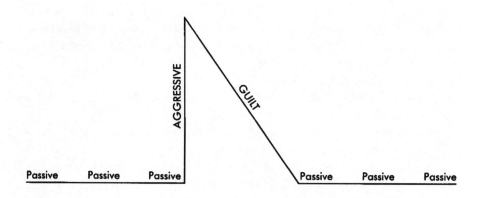

To interrupt this self-defeating cycle, it is necessary to convert many of the passive encounters into assertive ones. That way there is no mountainous buildup of minor incidents, and an emotional avalanche is prevented.

If after any exchange you feel used, guilty, angry, stupid, hurt, violated, or destroyed, then you have been the victim of aggression. If after any exchange the other person experiences these feelings, then you have been the aggressor.

It is vital to remember that a manipulator needs a manipulatee. When you start refusing to be manipulated, the other person is bound to be somewhat disappointed, irritated, or inconvenienced, but that is a far cry from being violated or destroyed.

Do not make the mistake of letting every turkey trot all over you until you lose control and try to make hash out of all of them at once. The secret of success is to tackle one turkey at a time. Try this for your meditation chant: "One turkey at a time . . . one turkey at a time . . . one turkey at a time."

Here are some examples given by women in the health professions. Their situations may sound all too familiar to you.

Turkey 1

Getting stuck with lots of personally meaningless activities is the most common complaint of women who fail to be assertive.

> "I just let someone assign me to another committee in an organization, when I'm already doing my share. I should have been assertive and said, 'No, thank you, but I can't help out on that committee at this time.' Instead I'm doing the extra job, but I'm not happy with myself about it! It's no one's fault but my own! My lack of assertiveness springs from a lack of self-confidence."

This woman had an excellent assertive response but did not use it. Or, if she did use it, she was not convincing. Refusing effectively takes practice. Be firm. If you waver, you will probably end up with the extra assignment.

Resist the urge to make excuses for refusing. It is difficult to invent convincing excuses on the spot, and most women feel guilty if they lie. However, the penalty for telling the truth—that there is no compelling reason for you to refuse the task—is to be given the chore.

Stick with the concrete theme: "No . . . not at this time." Repeat it as often as necessary.

Turkey 2

"The reason I am calling you is that I am handicapped. . . ."

This preamble is a telephone solicitor's way of trying to sell you everything from rug cleaners to candles, greeting cards to light bulbs. The word "handicapped" is meant to trigger feelings of sympathy and guilt. Whenever the flags of sympathy and guilt begin flying, beware! You are about to be manipulated.

After a brief introductory appeal, there is usually a pause in which they ask if they may now read through a list of products to see if you would be interested in any of them. This is where I say, "No, thank you, I am not interested in purchasing anything today, but thank you for calling. Goodbye." I learned to do this the hard way. I have a cupboard full of household products that cost twice as much as name-brand items and work half as well.

Saying no to random hits for money is often difficult. After all, how can you refuse someone less fortunate than yourself? Politely. You refuse politely.

Women in the health professions have deep-rooted needs to help others. If you do not want to become bitter and burned out, it is essential to designate who these others are. You are only human. Your resources are limited. The assertive response is to seek out individuals and organizations with which you want to share your resources.

Turkey 3

"Our pastor said I should tell my daughter that he wouldn't love her anymore if she didn't join the junior choir. Luckily, I came up with the statement that I couldn't do that because it sounded too unchristian. His request still bothers me, and I have great difficulty going to his service. I've seen him being manipulative at church meetings."

Whether the person is a pastor, scientist, administrator, or professor, each is human. Each has a NOT OK. Some handle the NOT OK in a healthy manner, and some do not.

We want to be perfect. We want others to be perfect, too—especially those in positions of authority. When they fail to be perfect, we may be sad or furious. At first, we may deny their imperfection and continue to follow faithfully. Even when the evidence is overwhelming, it is difficult to denounce a person whose position you have been taught to respect or revere.

Trust your feelings, intuition, and experience. Do not put your trust in degrees, rank, or position. A turkey is a turkey, even if he wears a clerical collar.

Turkey 4

"I worked with one nurse's aide who never seemed to be able to get her work done. She was always making excuses and getting somebody to help her, no matter how light her work load was for the day.

I always tried to cover for her, because she said she needed the job so badly. So I would give her easy patients. But one day she even had me helping her with bed-making! I was so mad at myself, I blew up and told her I just couldn't cope with her excuses."

Many marginal people seem to be attracted to less-skilled jobs in the health professions. Blinded by huge needs of their own, they find it nearly impossible to deal with patient needs. Women in the health professions are more tolerant of these employees than private industry would be.

There is a lot of Mother Hen in all of us. We try to have a "therapeutic" relationship with everyone. Our rescue needs spill over from patients onto co-workers, family, neighbors, and strangers. We are good listeners, patient, forgiving, and long-suffering. We are suckers for a hard-luck story.

Time after time, inadequate employees add to our burden, infuriate fellow workers, and lower the quality of patient care, but we feel a responsibility to carry them, to cover for them. We give and give and give, while they take and take and take. When we are mentally, emotionally, and physically exhausted, we explode. There is an angry tirade, and afterward we feel guilty. We want to minimize their shortcomings, make excuses for their behavior, and give them another chance, thus perpetuating a miserable situation.

When an employee fails to do her fair share of work, it is important to intervene long before the situation becomes critical. Begin collecting data when the problem is first noticed. Keep a record of the number of tasks she did and did not finish, the number and content of excuses given, the times late for work, times absent, and errors made. Then sit down with the employee privately and describe the situation in detail.

In working with psychiatric patients, it is often said that you will get the behavior you expect. If you expect them to be bizarre and violent, they will not disappoint you. Similarly, if you expect your employee to be late, slow, inefficient, and helpless, that is certainly the behavior you will get.

Take a bold, confident, positive approach: "This is what I expect. Let's try it out for a week and see how it goes." Help her set goals and do some problem solving, but resist the temptation to adopt her or her problems as your own.

After a week or two, sit down and reevaluate what you see happening. Praise her for achievements. However, if the problem persists, tell her frankly that she is simply not working out and that you intend to recommend she be dismissed.

There may be crying, pleading, or swearing, but through it all you must keep your eye on the patient's best interest. You are responsible for the patient's comfort and safety. Do not confuse the work relationship with a therapeutic relationship.

Turkey 5

"I was late for a class as a student nurse because I had duties to finish in the recovery room. The instructor was most unkind in her remarks and embarrassed me in front of my classmates. I would have liked to have told her my thoughts and reasons for being tardy but felt insecure and somewhat inferior—since she was the teacher."

Once again, we have the problem of inferior people in superior positions. Insecure instructors need to keep students ever mindful of their subordinate role. This instructor was rude. At the very least, she deserves a BM sticker.

Whenever you are treated unjustly, do not suffer silently. Face the instructor after class and say: "I felt very embarrassed and angry when you made those remarks about my being late. I would like to give you the reasons for my behavior now if you would be willing to listen."

If you are afraid of repercussions from openly sharing your feelings with the instructor, let off steam in a less direct way—smack a tennis ball, jog, write a letter detailing your feelings and then destroy it, or share your humiliation with a good friend who will listen. Whatever you do, do not swallow your feelings. They will make you sick.

Please savor and remember the humiliations you've endured as a student or a subordinate. When you arrive at the superior position, do not do unto others as you have been done unto.

Turkey 6

"A patient was emotionally ill and was hospitalized in a general hospital. She had physical symptoms caused by her emotional illness. Every time her husband came, she became upset, short of breath, and extremely nervous. Then her husband would hassle us about getting the doctor to come and see her immediately. When the doctor was contacted, he would chuckle, make off-hand remarks about her nerves, and let us handle the upset husband.

If I had it to do over again, I would have referred the doctor to the psychiatrist! I would have also pointed out to the husband what effect he was having on his wife. Maybe it wouldn't have helped anyone, but I would have felt better about the whole situation."

The doctor's mobility is indeed enviable. He can leave for surgery, his office, another unit, or the golf course, but the nurse is confined to the immediate situation. She is left holding the bag literally and figuratively.

Again, your actions should be guided by the best interest of the patient. Obviously, in this situation, she is not being helped. Document on the chart what you see happening, including the telephone calls to the doctor and his responses. Telephone the doctor, and when you get him on the line, hand the phone to the husband. Try to make sure the husband's visit coincides with the doctor's rounds at least once.

This is one of the many times when it is handy to have a psychiatrist willing to consult with your staff. If a psychiatrist is not available to you, get organized and petition the administration for this sort of consulting service. Pester them until you get it.

If this were my situation, I would probably speak to the wife alone about my observations. For example:

"I've noticed something kind of interesting, and I was wondering if you had noticed it, too. During the day, you seem relaxed and at ease. But after supper, when your husband arrives, you get short of breath and seem very nervous. Is that the way it seems to you, too?"

She may be relieved to have the obvious put into words, and a torrent of hopes and fears may tumble out. She may be furious and leave the hospital in a huff. Either way, hearing those words from a professional source may make her more accepting of future psychiatric treatment.

Turkey 7

Whoever said, "Sticks and stones may break my bones, but words can never hurt me," was wrong. I have not seen any women in the health professions battered physically, but I have seen many who were scared and scarred by words. Being sensitive to others is one of our strengths, but it also leaves us very vulnerable to verbal abuse.

"While I was working the 3 to 11:30 shift one evening, a doctor began shouting at me for something that had happened during the day shift. The fact that I hadn't been in the hospital at the time of the incident didn't seem to matter to him. There are many things I wish I had had the nerve to tell him."

Women tend to personalize verbal attacks. Even though this nurse knows she is not responsible for the incident, she feels some guilt by association. The error was made on this unit; this is my unit; therefore, I am guilty. This is the logical illogic that makes many women shoulder shame and blame for events beyond their control.

The passive response is to feel sad or depressed or to smolder silently. The aggressive response is to shout back at the doctor and usually feel angry with yourself afterward for losing control. The assertive response is to speak up. After the doctor finishes shouting, tell him calmly: "I can see you are upset (concerned, furious, whatever), but I was not present at the time of the event. However, I would be willing to work with you to make matters right."

Whenever you encounter someone with a verbal hemorrhage like this doctor, there are all sorts of actions you can take:

- Walk away. Taking verbal abuse is not in your job description.
- Wait until the doctor takes a breath (they have to breathe), and interject, "YES!" with great enthusiasm. It is distracting. They expect you to say, "NO, NO, NO!" They pause, trying to figure out why you are agreeing with them.
- Drop to one knee and cry, "Don't hit me!" This really discombobulates them. They back off, imploring, "Get up—don't do that!"
- In assertiveness training classes the importance of direct eye contact is always stressed. This may be the one exception. Do not look the doctor in the eye. Stare at his mouth. Soon he will realize he is verbally out of control. Even better, he begins to wonder if he has spinach stuck in his teeth.

And, my personal favorite:

- Lean forward and say, "Have a breath mint." It totally destroys the abuser.

Learning to speak up to authorities is a major hurdle for women in the health professions. One nurse was working on a neonatal unit when three babies in critical condition were transferred in at the same time. Staffing was poor, and she had only a licensed practical nurse to help her. The doctor was very nervous and demanding. At one point, she simply turned to him and said, "I only have two hands; just tell me what you want done first." He smiled and was much more understanding then.

Another crusty old physician had the irritating habit of talking down to the nursing staff. He kept making snide remarks, as though he thought the staff was planning to destroy all the good he intended to do. Finally, one nurse spoke up: "Look, Dr. K, I care just as much about Mrs. C as you do—perhaps even more. I intend to do everything in my power to help her get well." After that confrontation, he mellowed considerably and continued to seek out that particular nurse to work with whenever possible.

Turkey 8

"Six RNs, six student nurses, four LPNs, and three aides left at 3:30, leaving me with one LPN and two aides to care for 23 patients, four of whom could be listed in poor condition (the rest were children under age 11). At the stroke of 4, one of the not-poor patients began hemorrhaging and was clinically in shock. His doctor was not in the house, nor could I get through to his clinic (busy line). I was calling from the room phone. On my way out of the room to get more dressings and Ace bandages, I told the LPN to call the emergency room doctor. Just at that moment, the head nurse came off the elevator from a meeting. The emergency room doctor and the attending doctor came within moments, and the boy was rushed to the operating room for resuturing of severed leg arteries. (The emergency room doctor had obtained x-rays and had started an IV before the attending doctor got there.)

After the boy was in the operating room, my head nurse told me I must never call 'just any doctor while the attending doctor is in his office,' nor should I 'ever let an LPN call a doctor when the symptoms require an RN to interpret them,' and that this was not a 'Blue Code' situation, so calling the emergency room doctor from his department was wasteful of his time.

I am afraid I totally lost my temper and quite literally yelled at her, 'I wish it had been an arrest—I know CPR!—but if he bleeds to death, I have nothing!' And I stammered and stuttered about this being an example of her poor staffing techniques . . . and I'm only one person. . . . It makes me mad all over again!"

Women frequently complain about supervisors and head nurses with Victorian attitudes and antiquated rule books. Years ago, nurses got the starch out of their uniforms, but some can't seem to get it out of their minds. You know the type: the head nurse who would interrupt mouth-to-mouth resuscitation to have you pick up the linen off the floor.

Many nurses report working in situations with criminal under-staffing. We have become accustomed to making do. We keep plugging holes in the dike, never facing the fact that a flood is inevitable. We always hesitate a little too long, until an emergency or disaster forces action. Allowing 1.67 nurses for 30 patients may look fine on budget sheets, but, when translated into people instead of percentages, it may fall short.

In this situation, the staff nurse did act in the best interest of her patient. The fact that recalling the incident makes her mad all over again means that there has never been proper resolution. The emotional explosion on the scene did not clear the air. Instead of fuming and festering in silence, the nurse should speak up again. This time, it would be better to choose a more neutral occasion and place, and to approach the head nurse privately:

"When that boy began bleeding and I could not reach his doctor, I was tense and frightened. He was in shock. I knew I had to work fast. I felt hurt and angry that you chose those moments to scold me. I think we have some serious staffing problems here, and I would like to help work out a more satisfactory arrangement.

The head nurse's criticism was ill timed. When emotions are running high, resist the urge to criticize. At times like this, the staff needs support. Stand up for them. Stand behind them. A comment that tells the staff nurse you realize what she had just gone through will go a long way in defusing emotions. For example: "You must have been awfully concerned about the boy. It is so frustrating not to be able to reach the right doctor during an emergency."

If there is reason to be upset about the way an emergency situation has been handled, wait for a more neutral time to correct any errors in procedure. Get the staff together and review policies. Help them do some problem solving, so that the next time difficulties arise, things will go more smoothly.

Turkey 9

"I am president of my local nurses' union. One of the nurses who works the midnight shift would start attacking me whenever she saw me. She would whine and complain: 'My union doesn't do anything for me. The secretaries in my husband's office make more than we do! Our union dues are too high.' However, this nurse never came to a union meeting or offered to help with anything.

So I decided to try to respond assertively instead of aggressively. One night when she was complaining again, I said, 'Norma, you have so many good ideas for our new contract that I'm going to put you on our negotiations committee. You will be a big asset at the meetings.'

Needless to say, she did not serve on the committee or start coming to the meetings, but at least she stopped complaining and whining to me."

What a wonderful response! The union representative called the turkey's bluff in a very bold, confident, positive manner. Instead of allowing Norma to continue describing the problem, she insisted she become part of the solution. Turkeys often need to be challenged to put up or shut up.

"I worked a full shift at the hospital. I had to skip lunch because we had an emergency at work. After work, I went to visit my stepfather, who was in the hospital, having recently suffered a stroke.

When I got home, I was greeted by my boyfriend and six of his hunting and drinking buddies. They asked me to light up the barbeque and defrost a couple of steaks. I asked them politely where their girlfriends and wives were. I was told they were at home because it was 'the boys' night out!' So I asked them to leave and 'go out.'"

It's time to try your own hand at telling a turkey to stuff it. Read the following situation. Try to imagine yourself standing at the doorway. Picture your own hospital administrator and his office.

Broken appointment

You stand at the door of the hospital administrator's office and knock lightly: "Excuse me, but I believe I have a 3 o'clock appointment with you."

The administrator glances up from his desk and says, "I'm too busy to see you today." He looks down at his desk and begins shuffling papers.

How would you respond?

1. Physical response (specifically, what happens to your body in such situations—perspire, sigh, palpitations, weak knees, etc.):

   _____

2. Emotional response (fear, anger, frustration, humiliation, etc.):

   _____

3. Verbal response:
   a. What I would like to say to him is "_____

   _____."

b. But, a more effective thing to say would be "_____

_____."

Setting up situations in this format has proved helpful in working with both large and small groups. A written exercise gives each person an opportunity to actively describe her feelings, have the fun of "telling the turkey off," and then settle down to the most important task: articulating a response that will keep communication open without compromising her position.

After everyone has had time to complete the exercise, ask for volunteers to call out "one word that describes something that happens to you physically" and then "one emotion you would experience as you stood at the door." What a relief to discover you are not alone! Others clench, tremble, blush, cry. Others feel sad, put down, outraged, humiliated.

Most are delighted to share their snappy comebacks under "What I would like to say is '_____.'" The responses are hilarious, and laughter is a great tension releaser.

After the giggles subside, the group settles down to the difficult task of forming words and selecting actions that communicate effectively. Be prepared for Freudian slips and lapses into passive or aggressive behavior. Although there is never one "right" answer, it will be obvious to the group that some choices are better than others. They will quickly chime in with variations, suggestions, or modifications. Help them look for responses that are confident, positive, brief, task centered, and non-threatening enough to invite further communication. Help them focus on I-messages instead of you-messages.

None of the situations in this book is fabricated. All have come from workshop participants. Please feel free to use any of them when working in a classroom or workshop setting. You will soon discover, however, that each group is teeming with examples of its own. You would be wise to take a few moments and let the participants write a description of a situation (personal or professional) in which they were assertive or *wish* they had been more assertive.

To help ensure anonymity, give them scratch paper and tell them not to sign their names. If the situation described is a sensitive one that would embarrass the writer or another group member, have these persons put a large star at the top of the page to indicate that it should not be shared. On the other hand, if they have a situation they would love to have analyzed or role-played, have them print "PLEASE USE" in large letters at the top of the page. Using situations that come directly from the group enables everyone to become more personally involved and gives the group a greater sense of accomplishment when they reach a solution.

Top turkey award

"As a clinical audiologist I had the unhappy experience of working for a doctor who often did more damage than good. I almost hated to tell patients their hearing loss was remediable by surgery when I worked in his office.

While I was checking a patient after surgery, he reported being able to detect some sounds better but said he was having a lot more trouble understanding speech. I explained that the results of the audio test indicated that hearing had improved slightly for low frequencies but had been reduced at higher frequencies, from a moderate conductive loss to a severe/profound sensorineural loss.

Then the doctor saw the patient and proceeded to lie. He said the patient's hearing had improved and was much better than before surgery.

The patient protested. He told the doctor that he was having much more difficulty understanding what was said to him. When the patient told the doctor that I had explained that his hearing was better only for some frequencies, the doctor blew a gasket. He exploded at me and said I was never to interpret an audio test for a patient again.

Naturally, the doctor was worried about being sued. However, he would have stood a much better chance of getting out of hot water with his wallet intact if he had told the patient preoperatively that surgery was a gamble (which it certainly was with this doctor!) and then had been honest with the patient about the results afterward.

I have known many competent surgeons who were very honest with their patients about surgical results. One excellent surgeon told his patient that surgery was unsuccessful and that he was sorry it had happened to such a nice person.

As a clinical audiologist, I am trained to interpret results. I was not overstepping my bounds. That patient could have gone to any audiologist in the state to be evaluated and counseled about surgical results.

After this incident I felt I had to make a decision. Could I stand behind a doctor who would lie about the results obtained with my skills? I found myself in a position where he couldn't tolerate my honesty and I couldn't tolerate giving tacit approval by remaining silent about the test findings. I decided there was no resolution to this problem. I told him my feelings, and I quit. Some situations are irresolvable and warrant resignation—the quitting kind.

I'm still angry about this, and the more experience I gain, the angrier I get."

This example makes me feel more strongly than ever that women in the health professions should collaborate and publish a directory of recommended physicians and facilities. Obviously, this turkey would not make the list.

. . .

Daily encounters with turkeys cannot be avoided. Your best defense is to value yourself, your time, and your resources. When you learn to do that, saying no will be less painful and saying yes will be a pleasure. When turkeys get the best of you and you blow up, do not brood or punish yourself. Just take the experience as a reminder to tackle one turkey at a time. Most important, do not swallow your feelings and opinions. Learn to speak up. "Let's talk, turkey."

8

Peacocks

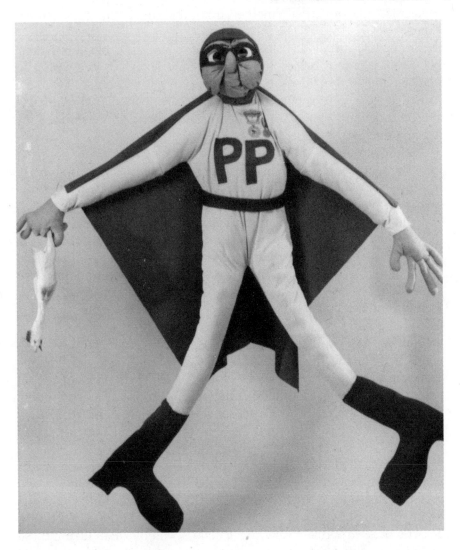

Patient protector.

Look—up in the air! It's a bird! It's a plane! No—it's PATIENT PROTECTOR!

Patient Protector—idol of the infirm, champion of the weak, defender of dignity.

Who would believe that in real life Patient Protector is just a mild-mannered health care worker? But at the first sign of patient distress, this quick-change artist emerges from the linen closet as Patient Protector!

Stunningly attired in a jaundice-yellow jumpsuit, blood-red cape, bile-green belt and mask, and cyanotic-blue boots, Patient Protector perches atop the patient's bed, scrutinizing all who enter the room. Armed only with a rubber chicken and a little legal Latin, Patient Protector defends patients from the high and the mighty, as well as the low and the loathsome.

Patient Protector—able to translate medical mumbo jumbo faster than the speed of sound, able to leap across to the corner drugstore for cheap aspirin and Kleenex, able to fetch a burger and fries when the hospital sends up creamed liver and banana casserole.

Who dares tackle tiresome visitors and tacky technicians? Who dares stump students who have neglected to do their homework? Who forces dietitians to down their own concoctions? Who heckles head nurses, interrogates interns, and razzes residents? Who waddles down the hall behind pompous physicians, quacking all the way? Who? Patient Protector!

Although most would agree that Patient Protector would be nothing without such an outlandish uniform, we are reluctant to accept the cliché that "clothes make the man." We have an aversion to thinking that something as superficial as clothing can have such impact. It makes people seem so shallow. After all, image is only a reflection. Image has no substance. It's what's inside that counts. But advertisers will tell you "it's what's up front that counts"; according to motivational researcher John T. Molloy, image is all that counts.

Molloy is billed as an "image engineer," and he has research results to show that how you decorate yourself and your surroundings can spell the difference between success and failure. In his initial study, he found that students worked harder and more conscientiously for teachers who dressed formally than for teachers who did not. Taking these findings, he quit teaching and launched a highly profitable career as writer, researcher, and consultant to individuals and companies seeking success.

Molloy suggests that doctors who follow his advice about wardrobes and waiting rooms are supposed to attract patients who pay bills promptly and don't bother them outside of office hours. He recommends a very restricted range of suits, shirts, ties, and shoes to be worn, adding such fine details as *always* having a leather band on your expensive but unostentatious watch.

In the ground-breaking books concerning image and success, only a few paragraphs were devoted to women. Models in the illustrations usually wore highly tailored, thick tweed suits, complete with shirt and tie. The visual message: Dress like a man. Perhaps the paucity of material available for women is what inspired Molloy to eventually write *The Woman's Dress for Success Book.*

In very condensed form, the rules say powerful, successful women will shun anything feminine or fashionable. They will be clothed in very tailored, dark-colored suits, shod with dark-colored leather pumps, and capped with maroon fedoras with a little feather. Polyester knits look cheap, so they are a no-no. Since handbags frighten men, successful women will carry only expensive leather briefcases, and they will sign everything with gold pens.

Where does all of this leave you and me? Hundreds of thousands of us are wearing white polyester knits with orthopedic shoes, sporting Timexes on Twist-o-Flexes, carrying enema cans instead of briefcases, and flicking our Bics. Nothing about us communicates success or power. In fact, our attire hardly distinguishes us from any waitress in an all-night diner.

One nurse from the East Coast reported shopping in a major department store whose uniform section was marked "NURSES AND OTHER DOMESTICS." Molloy says, "If you dress like a vice president, you will be treated like a vice president." It would logically follow that if you dress like a domestic, you will be treated like a domestic. When discussing image and the woman health professional, one nurse summed it up this way: "Most of the time, I feel I am invisible."

Being invisible does have its advantages. It is safer to blend into the background. You will most likely be left alone. Many women are content to just float along as another forgettable face amid an endless sea of white. They are content until they want to call attention to a problem or make changes in patient care policy.

That's when being invisible puts you at a terrible disadvantage. You are so easy to ignore. You are totally forgettable. People with power to make changes may appear to listen but not take you seriously enough to act on your suggestions. You have no muscle. There are no threats you can enforce. They know if they stall temporarily, you will just drift away into the background. The system remains unchanged.

It would be nice if powerful people cared more about issues than images, but it may be naive to think they do. The powerful are very image-oriented. Their main concern is making sure everything looks good—especially on paper. Why else would medical institutions need public relations departments? Instead of expensive PR campaigns designed to whitewash problems and keep institutions looking good, let's work on solving the problems and making institutions better. A staff that is proud of their institution and confident of the care they give has little need for a public relations department.

Although it may seem vain and foolish to put too much emphasis on outward appearance, it is equally foolhardy to put too little emphasis on it. Plumage is important. Molloy calls the physician's short white jacket "the most powerful authority symbol in the world."

The authority conveyed by a doctor's duds can be illustrated by an amusing incident that occurred in July 1981 at John Peter Smith Hospital in Fort Worth.

During a power failure late one stormy Friday night, a young man dressed in a scrub suit stepped forward and took command of the situation. With the temperature soaring and no air-conditioning available, he dispatched the staff on a late-night expedition to gather ice. They wound up with 2000 pounds of ice in the hospital lobby. That was only one of his many *accomplishments* during the crisis.

It wasn't discovered until the wee hours of Sunday morning that the "doctor" was really a patient on the hospital's unlocked psychiatric ward.

At last we have a solution for women health professionals who don't want to be confused with the domestic staff: simply wear a short white coat or a scrub suit. Instant respect. Instant authority. Instant power.

Well-known image consultant Roger Ailes, author of *You Are the Message,* suggests you have seven seconds to communicate who and what you are. *Seven* seconds.

If you approach a patient in a flowered top, with Mickey Mouse underwear showing through tight, white pants, your appearance does not say, "I am a professional. Put your life in my hands." It says, "For a good time call Bobbie Jo." And then Bobbie Jo wonders why she doesn't get any respect.

Instead of focusing on dress codes, which tends to set everyone's teeth on edge, we need to focus on the image we are projecting to patients and their families. Think about it. Would you board an airplane where the pilot and crew dressed as randomly and carelessly as many hospital workers do?

Although sex therapists tell people to strip and stand naked in front of full-length mirrors, if you want to see something really revealing, try dressing for work and then standing in front of a full-length mirror. Like it or not, the clothes you wear say something about you. Among nonverbal messages, clothing speaks first. What are your clothes saying?

"I am casual."

"I am careless."

"I am professional."

"I have money."

"I am sexy."

"I had spaghetti for lunch."

Professionals in the psychiatric setting were the first to move out of uniforms and into street clothes. At one point, it was feared the staff might be competitive in trying to outdress each other. Almost the reverse occurred. Molloy stresses the importance of keeping business and leisure clothes separate. Leisure clothes say things like "Relax" or "Why work?" or "Don't take me too seriously." It might be interesting to speculate on whether the staff members' clothing compounds verbal and nonverbal messages enough to confuse patients and impede therapy.

The pediatric setting is another place where uniforms have been abandoned in favor of calico frocks that might have been designed by Mother Surrogate. I supported such changes until my own 4-year-old was confronted by a pediatric resident dressed like a calypso dancer. Eric eyed him suspiciously. When the resident tried to examine him, Eric squirmed and screamed. I was alarmed, because he had never been afraid of doctors or dentists before.

When a doctor with a white jacket entered the room, Eric calmed down quickly and cooperated happily. I left wondering whether abandoning uniforms was really such a good idea. As simple-minded as it may sound, it is comforting to be able to tell the "good guys" from the "bad guys" by their garb. Instead of making children afraid of white uniforms, we may just be fostering a calico phobia.

The uniform–versus–street clothes quandary makes me think of the effect my uniform had on me when I was a student. I felt I had two distinct identities. Around the dormitory, I wore sloppy clothes and engaged in general silliness. My behavior and attitudes changed abruptly when I put on the starched white cap and uniform to go to the hospital. Technically still a teenager, I was initially surprised by the way patients bared not only their bodies but their souls. People two, three, or four times my age looked to me for comfort and guidance. My clothes made an enormous difference in the way people responded to me and, even more dramatically, in the way I responded to them.

Clothing does have a communication all its own. The next time you go to the hospital cafeteria, look around and see what wordless messages you can pick up. Wanting to display some external evidence of worth or expertise is normal. Watch for name tags with impressive titles, badges, buttons, pipes, beards, lab coats, a smattering of surgical chic, and students who conspicuously adorn their bodies with stethoscopes. (If you've got it, flaunt it!) A humorous article on the pecking order in the hospital was printed in *The Atlantic* 35 years ago. Even though nurses' uniforms have changed in many institutions during the past three decades, this article is still fresh and delightful today:

HOSPITAL HIERARCHY*

Marjorie Taubenhaus

In any modern hospital a pecking order, similar to that seen in bird flocks, may be observed. Of course, differences between birds and hospitals exist. Birds determine precedence simply and quickly upon meeting. They fight. The stronger bird gains for all time the right to peck the weaker. The human beings involved in a hospital situation are accustomed to use symbols as surrogates for physical combat. These symbols are usually expressed as degrees, such as M.D., R.N., or M.Sc. However, like people, once birds have established their relative rank, a peculiar, often sonorous sound, called the threat sound, may be used to maintain superiority relationships.

There is one important point of differentiation between the bird and hospital pecking orders. It lies in the ability of the birds to recognize one another. People have had to develop elaborate systems of insignia and dress to ensure the recognition of rank that is intuitively grasped by birds. The confusing multiplicity of uniforms observed in any hospital is readily understood if we know that a three hundred to four hundred bed hospital may have about a thousand persons engaged directly or indirectly with the care of patients and the running of the hospital. Most bird flocks are not this complex. The variety of dress provides a

---

*From *The Atlantic*, vol. 203, June 1959. Copyright © 1959, by The Atlantic Monthly Company, Boston, Mass. Reprinted with permission.

clue to the pecking order and not a functional guide for the casual visitor to the hospital.

Top man on the hospital pecking pole is the doctor. He has invested at least eight years of his life in college and medical school for the ultimate privilege of wearing a long, loose white coat. No belt in the back, it flops freely in the breeze as the physician autocratically strides down the hospital corridors. Some lucky few in every hospital wear coats threadbare and out at the elbows; these are the chiefs of service. Brown-edged acid holes, however, denote only research workers. These command no special respect except in those obscure, rarefied circles where Nobel is more than a synonym for aristocratic.

Between the long white coat and the white-jacketed medical student (stethoscope peeping coyly from his pocket) stand the intern and resident. These wear white trousers, white jackets, and white shirts, hospital issue. This costume entitles the wearer to full respect on the wards, tolerance in the semiprivate rooms, and outraged demands for a doctor from the private suites.

Although the registered nurse may not have worked through as many schools as the doctor, she has undoubtedly worked through a great many more uniforms. She achieves the final triumph of the dress-that-stands-by-itself only after progressing through the blue of the student, doffing an apron here, and picking up a cap there. Very often black lines are added to her cap and extra pins to her dress at specified and very special milestones along the way. When she has finally graduated, with the frilly headpiece chosen by the hospital of her training (as its own announcement to the world that "This nurse does things the way we do") she is then officially qualified to say "yes" to a doctor's face and "no" behind his back to everybody else in the world. The maid, the aide, the intern in his first months of training, all must turn their cheek to her peck. They may draw small comfort from the knowledge that half the starch in her uniform probably comes from the dressing down the staff doctor has just given her.

The orderly relationships of the nursing echelons are probably the most clearly defined of any in the hospital and are reflected in a veritable rainbow array of uniforms. The trained practical nurse wears white, but without a registered nurse pin, and her consequent lack of authority to dispense medications leaves her not a social leg to stand on. The student is not only in blue and white, but for the first six months of her training she is bareheaded. Once she is capped, she is well on her way up the ladder. The nurse's aide may be in green, the orderly in tan, and who can forget the Grey Lady? Order of precedence is firmly established in these variations of color and form, and a whole organization of supervisors and directors exists to protect it.

Many large urban hospitals today have social service departments, realistically as well as self-consciously important in the framework of twentieth-century medical care. On the wards the medical social worker wears a white coat, her department identified only by a nameplate on the lapel and the oddity of the coiffure above. The social worker ranks herself ostensibly just below the physician, but in truth is answerable only to God and the psychiatrist.

The hospital chef wears white in well-respected, nonmedical tradition, but he has been outmaneuvered by the dietitians. In most restaurants and hotels all over the world the high white hat of the cook represents the acme of dictatorial prestige. But the hospital dietitians have pre-empted this authority as well as a nurse's uniform. Caught in a net of calories and low-residue diets, the chef's superiority to the green-clad dishwashers is small compensation for the pecks of the nutrition experts.

Laboratory technicians circulate through the hospital in stained white coats. At feud level with the nurses, they lack the magnificent hierarchical nursing organization. Some are experts in their own field, highly specialized and correspondingly trained. Some are just routine test runners. But the white coat covers a multitude of skills, and the technician title gives the right to a few pecks here and there.

Some few secretaries in a hospital have fought through a right to a white coat. They are the envied ones, even though they may have to suffer the slings and arrows of outrageous surgical chiefs for their dubious privilege. For, who knows? They may one day be taken for technicians.

The nether regions, both actual and rhetorical, are inhabited by a variety of persons and uniforms. Hospitals are fond of the term "ancillary personnel," and it includes the engineers, maintenance men, and laundry workers concealed in the hospital basement as well as the maids, elevator men, and pages.

The bottom of the pecking order is represented by its own, peculiarly humiliating uniform. The hospital patient, outranked by the lowliest pantrywoman, is exposed literally and figuratively in a short white chemise. This garment, barely reaching to mid-thigh, is split the length of the back and inadequately fastened at the neck and waist with strings. If a patient thinks that his position as Chairman of the Board of twenty-two large industries gives him any status, his hospital gown is calculated to dispel the delusion.

Aside from clothing, there are other nonverbal aspects that can either enhance or inhibit your attempts to be assertive. If you want to be assertive, it is nice to be tall. If you aren't tall, standing up straight will help. Posture is important. The way you carry yourself says a lot about you.

Eye contact is crucial. Keep your head up, and look the other person in the eye. If you bow your head or keep averting your eyes, your message loses much of its impact.

Body language can give you away. Nervous movements, such as swinging your foot, playing with rings, twisting your hair, biting your lip, squirming, or fidgeting, can undo your efforts to present a bold, confident, positive front. Keep hands quiet and relaxed. Don't clench or clutch.

Often it is not what you say but how you say it that counts. Stammering or groping for words does not reflect boldness. A timid, weak voice does not communicate confidence. A shrill, whining, or nagging tone can drive people away in droves. To be assertive, you need a full, well-modulated voice. Choose words carefully, and speak clearly.

Whatever the message, thought, or feeling you wish to convey to others, remember the three watchwords: bold, confident, and positive. State what you have to say frankly and concisely. Let the listener judge the content of the message independently. Don't try to prejudge, qualify, or compromise your message during delivery.

Armed with all this information, how would you handle the following situation?

A few weeks ago three of you were selected to attend your national professional convention at the hospital's expense. Not only does the convention program promise to be highly informative, it will take place in Hawaii. Hawaii! You've dreamed of going there for years.

This morning you learned that budget cutbacks mean there will be enough funding to send only one person to the convention. You desperately want to be the one chosen to go.

Sell yourself as the best candidate.
1. List four to six phrases that will help "sell" you:

_____

_____

_____

_____

2. How will your behavior be affected if:
   a. The administrator interviews each of you separately before choosing?_____

_____

   b. The administrator meets with the three of you together?

_____

_____

3. How might you sabotage yourself? _____

_____

This is an excellent situation to role-play or assign as a group task. Every woman needs to realize that selling herself doesn't have to mean selling others out.

We are so conditioned to being polite and to putting others first that we often miss out on rare and wonderful opportunities. THE RIGHT TO ASK FOR WHAT YOU WANT is a most difficult one for women to accept. In fact, I have discovered that women hesitate to ask for what they *need,* let alone what they want.

A common error in communicating is to use negative phrasing. For example: "I don't suppose you can spare an extra nurse for our unit today." The underlying message delivered is that you really don't expect help, and therefore you probably won't receive it. It is also a mistake to preface comments with apologetic phrases, such as "This probably isn't very important, but . . ." or "I know you hate to be bothered, but. . . ." The underlying message is that the speaker is unimportant and a bother.

When you have an important confrontation coming up, it helps to plan and rehearse. You do not need to memorize a speech word for word, but try to think of alternate phrases that express your ideas effectively. This is where an assertiveness training group can be very helpful. If you don't have a group, ask an articulate friend to listen to your ideas and help you choose suitable words and phrases. Some find practicing in front of a mirror helpful.

Behavior speaks loudly. A mother who had roomed-in with her young child during a 2-week hospitalization made some interesting observations on the doctor-nurse relationship. While staying with her child all hours of the day and night, she came to know the nurses working on the unit very well. She was impressed by their wealth of knowledge and experience, their skillful guidance, and their excellent support of children and families through crises, including death. Her confidence in them grew daily, and she came to trust their judgment completely.

Because of the way she came to feel about the nurses, she found their behavior around the medical staff perplexing and irritating. Whenever the medical staff arrived, usually in bunches, the nurses would stop in the middle of whatever they were doing and retreat to a corner of the room to stand silently while the doctors talked among themselves. Rarely did the nurses volunteer information or comment on what they thought might be helpful. It was rarer still for the doctors to seek their opinions.

This quiet withdrawing of women whom she considered highly skilled and intelligent baffled her. She vividly recalled an incident when one of the doctors dropped his pen and a nurse quickly knelt to pick it up. This example seemed to sum up what she had observed over the 2 weeks. She left vowing her daughter would never be a nurse.

Even though nurses have gotten away from standing when a doctor enters the room, the groveling reflex is still strong. Nurses keep talking about a colleague relationship with physicians, but talk is cheap. What doctors and nurses do (how they interact or fail to interact) speaks more loudly than what they say. There can never be a colleague relationship between master and servant.

Keeping us ever mindful of our lesser station in life is the environment. Our surroundings send out subtle but continuous messages. Look at the various areas of your institution. You can assess the importance of the people occupying them by the amount of space, quality of furnishings, and depth of carpeting.

Have you ever been ushered into the doctors' conference room or the room where the board of directors meets once a month? The setting is plush. Contrast that with the conference space available to the bulk of hospital employees. Most women are grateful for a vacated broom closet. We are glad to have any space where we can spend a few uninterrupted moments discussing and planning patient care.

For an environmental message reflecting the institution's view of your value, go to the women employees' locker room. One interior decorator does hospital locker rooms nationwide. The walls are invariably painted with an unusual pastel shade somewhere between blah and yuck. The paint industry manages to mistakenly mix about 4000 gallons each year and then distributes it wholesale to institutions at twice what a normal color would cost. The furniture has all the warmth of cheap plastic and comes in a variety of gaudy colors accentuated by masking tape over splits and tears. Completing the decor are corroded plumbing fixtures and mosaic tile floors with random pieces missing. The atmosphere is enhanced by a heavy pine-scented disinfectant splashed liberally by the housekeeping department, whose members can barely tolerate being in the room long enough to do minimal upkeep. The room is a marvelous place to relax, take a break, converse with friends, and confer with colleagues.

Many nurses are still required to punch time clocks. This minor ritual keeps the nursing staff guessing about their professional status and chips away at any inflated idea they may have about their self-worth. The subtle implication is that management cannot trust nurses to do an honest day's work. Working with sick people, however, is not as predictable as assembly-line work, and overtime begins to pile up. Management regrets they cannot compensate for overtime but feels that the nursing staff—as a professional group—must realize patient care cannot be regulated by a clock. Confusing, isn't it?

Bombarded with put-downs from the environment and management, it is no wonder we have difficulty salvaging our self-esteem. Our attire, working conditions, salary, lack of access to policy-making boards, and pervasive powerlessness add up to a domestic image instead of a professional one.

Although the domestic image may be difficult to avoid, the domestic mentality—dull, plodding, unquestioning, subservient—is something women health professionals are finding easier to refuse. We are skilled. We are intelligent. We are the majority.

Early in his career the famous architect Frank Lloyd Wright said he had to choose between honest arrogance and hypocritical humility. He chose the former. Isn't it time we permitted ourselves a little honest arrogance and reveled in unabashed, unashamed appreciation of the talents, skills, and experiences that have made us the professionals we are today?

The time has come to make the silent majority visible. No more timid titmouse. It is a shame Patient Protector is just a figment of the imagination. We could use a role model with a dash more flair, imagination, and daring to help us shed the dowdy plumage assigned to those who are bland, conservative, and methodical.

Maybe we should all show up for work wearing Patient Protector costumes. Initially, the administration might mistake us for clowns, but they would soon learn that this is no laughing matter. Women constitute between 80 and 85 percent of the health service work force. We have the right to be recognized, to be taken seriously, and to share in making any decisions or policies that affect patient care or our jobs.

Image is an issue too long ignored by women in the health professions. As individuals we may be invisible, but if we were ever to unite, there would be a tidal wave on that subservient sea of white that could forever alter the present health care system, if not sweep it away entirely.

9

Pigeons

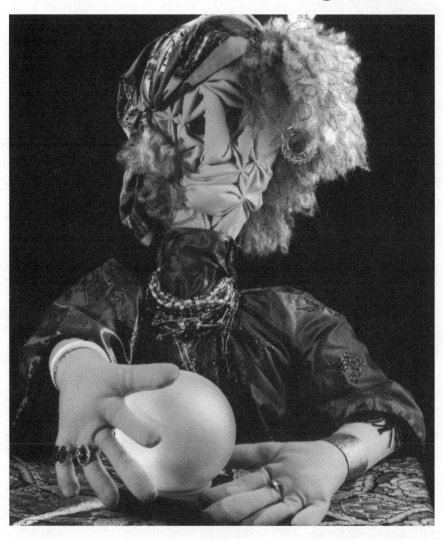

Want your fortune, Cookie?

To borrow and bend a phrase from P.T. Barnum, there's a pigeon born every minute, and at least half of them are women. Pigeons are people who are a little too naive, a little too gullible, a little too trusting.

For all the pigeons out there, I have some good news and some bad news. The bad news is that the world is full of manipulators, both malignant and benign. The good news is that people can only manipulate you if you let them. You can't blame a guy for trying. You have the option to say no.

> "We paid for our daughter's braces a year ago with a check marked paid in full. Two months ago, our orthodontist's bookkeeper informed me we owed several hundred dollars more because she wore the braces longer than planned.
>
> They called me at my job. I was shocked and unable to say anything except 'okay.' As the day passed and I continued to think about it, I decided this was crazy. I called and informed them no further payment would be made. I felt good!"

Although you are surrounded by people who are ready, willing, and able to take advantage of you, not all of them are malicious. Most of them are just trying to get a job done and see you as a means of accomplishing their task. This applies to the persistent potato-peeler salesman, as well as the parish priest.

Several times a day you may be tested to see how much work or worry you are willing to give to a cause. Like most women, you may be a giver, but after a while you tire of making sacrifices, doing extra duty, missing social functions, being expected to always come through in a pinch, and settling for a pat on the back instead of an increase in your paycheck.

When your sense of humor and sunny disposition begin to fade, you have given enough. The time has come to look at how your life is being spent. Are you spending your life, or is someone else always borrowing it and spending it for you?

For some people time is money. For all of us time is life. Unlike a cup of sugar, time borrowed can never be returned.

Look at those around you, and think about how you take advantage of them. If you want something done for you, how do you approach others? Think about the people you usually ask for favors. Someone quipped, "If you can't take advantage of your friends, whom can you take advantage of?"

Vacation

This year you have made elaborate plans for your vacation. Reservations were completed almost 3 months ago. You are eagerly counting the few remaining days until you leave. This morning you are called to your supervisor's office and told that the other head nurse on your floor has just resigned—effective immediately.

Supervisor: "I know your vacation was to begin Monday, but you can see what a terrible bind we're in! I hate to impose, but you are the only person who could possibly manage both units at once. Mary's resignation certainly was a shock—so irresponsible. I'm glad I've always been able to count on you."

How would you respond?

1. Physical response: _____

2. Emotional response: _____
3. Verbal response:
   a. What I would like to say to her is "_____

   _____."

   b. But, a more effective thing to say is "_____

   _____."

The best way to keep people from taking advantage of you and using your life is to be able to recognize the ploys likely to be used against you. Here are a few to consider.

Flattery. Women's work is so often taken for granted that you may not only be hungry for praise or recognition, you may be starving. It's hard to keep your head when a sweet talker comes along cooing, "You are the only person I can really talk to" or "You are the best nurse on the floor."

Whenever you find yourself being buttered up, beware: chances are you are about to be manipulated. Accept compliments graciously, but resist the compulsion to return a compliment or to comply with the flatterers' requests just because you want to keep their esteem. If their esteem is that shallow, it isn't worth keeping.

Criticism. This ploy is the opposite of flattery but just as effective. If flattery fails, criticism may quickly follow in its footsteps. Even a slight implication that you are a bad mother, an inadequate wife, or an insensitive therapist can cut you to the bone. All the NOT OK feelings suddenly surface. You begin to doubt yourself again. Perhaps you are not as wise or wonderful, as competent or compassionate as you thought. Perhaps you are being selfish or illogical.

Acceptance of your own nonperfect self is not a one-time conquest. You may have to deal with it again. Give yourself time to sort through critical remarks. Remember to consider their content and their intent. Consider the source. Do not make any long-range plans, sweeping changes in your lifestyle, or coerced commitments when you are feeling down on yourself.

Insecurity. A would-be manipulator makes good use of your fears. For example, the underlying fear that you can always be replaced may make you take on all kinds of extra tasks so that your family or employer will see how indispensable you are. Soon the extra tasks are absorbed into the standard expectations. To keep winning the irreplaceable title, you have to take on more and more tasks, until you buckle under the load.

> "Because of understaffing on the evening shift, we were not getting a supper break. This went on for 2 years, and we were too afraid to say anything. Then they tried to increase our work load. Enough! I went to the manager (fearfully) and explained the situation.
>
> She quickly found a remedy. A part-time person was hired to cover 5 to 9 PM. I can't believe we endured that situation for 2 years and the manager solved it in 2 days! Why didn't one of us speak up sooner?"

A mere hint that love is about to be withdrawn makes many women hastily comply with a manipulator's demands. If you are terrified at the prospect of being left alone, it is time you got to know yourself and like yourself better. Only then will you be able to withstand such a cowardly and cruel attack.

Fear of what people will think exerts a lot of control over your behavior. This fear keeps you searching for the straight and narrow road supposedly trod by good mothers, good wives, good neighbors, good customers, good therapists, good whatevers. Unfortunately, this road is so nebulous that even a good whatever is likely to have a nervous breakdown trying to follow it.

When anticipating how assertiveness will look on you, it is natural to ask, "What will people think?" The answer is simply: "People will think anything they please." You have no control over other people's thoughts. It is what you think that is important. Don't be too quick to alter your behavior on the basis of what people might think. Their thoughts are unpredictable.

Fear of offending someone—anyone!—keeps many women from

being assertive. If a manipulator is offended when you refuse to comply, just hum the line from the popular song that goes, "You can't please everyone, so you've got to please yourself."

Our insecurity gives manipulators excellent leverage to use against us. Insecurity can be highly profitable. For example, women have spent millions of dollars on feminine deodorant products that have been shown to be virtually useless and potentially harmful.

Have you ever wondered why dry cleaners charge more to do a woman's cotton blouse than a man's cotton shirt? Have you ever wondered why department stores charge women for alterations and yet will do extensive alterations for men at no charge? Women pay more than men for almost everything from cars to haircuts. It's all documented in a book titled *Why Pay More?* by Frances Cerra Whittelsey.*

Talk about pigeons—women are paid less and then charged more! But don't just get mad, get this book and then get even.

Your assignment for today is to think about the things you have done and the products you have purchased because you weren't secure enough to refuse or resist.

Helplessness. The old what-would-I-do-without-you routine capitalizes on your need to be needed. The corporate tycoon who can't straighten his tie or remember his appointments somehow manages to make millions. His secretary, like all other unsung heroines, is content to stay in the background, poor but secure in the knowledge that he couldn't do it without her.

Women often foster helpless behavior in others and then complain and condemn that same behavior. A husband may be all thumbs at cooking or cleaning; so the wife takes over those chores again. The husband sighs, "Well, I tried." The wife is again overworked but temporarily more content, because she has proved once again that he couldn't manage without her.

Resist the urge to rush in and take over someone else's work just because he or she appears helpless or because you know you can do it faster. All of us have strengths that outnumber our weaknesses. Husbands and children can be helpful instead of helpless. It just takes practice, patience, and praise.

Obligation. It's your duty as a citizen (nurse, mother, Christian) to do

---

*Available from the Center for Study of Responsive Law, P.O. Box 19367, Washington, D.C. 20036.

this, that, and the other thing. Women have been made to feel responsible for the welfare and happiness of others. That's a tall order. Ensuring welfare is difficult; ensuring happiness is impossible.

Obviously, you do have obligations to your husband, children, employer, and others. What is often overlooked is that these people also have obligations to you. Agreeing to share your life with others brings obligations that differ from those that accompany agreeing to give your life to others.

Parenthood brings obligations that seem to go on forever.

> "Our son dropped out of school and wasn't motivated to work or get out on his own. When we stopped giving him money, he finally found a job. He was a slob and expected me to clean up after him. He refused to help me or his father.
>
> All of a sudden, my husband gave him an ultimatum: he had 30 days to find an apartment and move out. To my surprise, it worked! Today he is on his own, feels successful, and is much happier."

This is an excellent example of the difference between helping and enabling. While their intentions were good, these parents were "enabling" their son to remain a bum. It wasn't until they cut off the easy money and kicked him out that they really "helped" him.

In our personal and professional lives we have to keep alert. It is easy to slip from helping to enabling. That's what codependence, one of the most popular topics in self-help literature, is all about. Definitions and descriptions of codependence vary widely, but one of my favorites is that it is a normal reaction to abnormal people. Codependence involves doing the wrong things for the right reasons.

For those of us in the helping professions, codependence is an occupational hazard. We spend our lives in close proximity to people who are troubled, needy, and dependent. We are only trying to help. Our intentions are good. But you know what they say, "The road to hell is paved with good intentions."

An alarm should go off when you find yourself:
- Doing something you don't want to do
- Saying yes when you mean no
- Meeting needs before being asked
- Doing more than your fair share
- Giving more than you receive
- Fixing other people's feelings
- Thinking for another person

• Suffering other people's consequences

• Failing to ask for what *you* need or want

These are just some of the signs that you are in a codependent relationship.

When you feel bogged down by things you "ought" to do or "should" do, rethink your priorities and obligations. You have no obligation to strive for sainthood or martyrdom. Martyrs are for burning.

Guilt. This sister of obligation is the ultimate weapon in the manipulator's arsenal. Feelings of guilt are powerful persuaders that are easily evoked and perhaps more difficult to deal with than any other emotion. Guilt is cunning, merciless, and usually Number One on the hit parade.

"It will break your mother's heart if you don't come home for Christmas."

"Thousands of people are starving to death, and you won't eat what's on your plate."

"You should be grateful just to be alive."

"If you really loved me, you would do as I ask."

"How can you refuse to help the poor and needy?"

Guilt comes in twinges and torrents. Whenever you begin feeling guilty, stop and examine what is happening to you. Guilt can become a way of life. Some women even feel guilty about feeling good.

When you are knee-deep in guilt, you are susceptible to all types of manipulation and may agree to do things as a form of self-punishment, a kind of penance for sins real or imagined. Wait for guilt to subside before making any agreements or commitments.

Georgia, a meticulously groomed woman in her sixties, always stopped by the cosmetics counter to see the latest beauty aids available. The clerk was delighted to show her something exciting and new. She sprayed a refreshing mist on Georgia's face and told her the product had just arrived and was already a best-seller.

Whenever you felt fatigued, you just sprayed the mist on your face and felt a wonderful uplift. The clerk assured Georgia it was completely natural and would act as an instant moisturizer.

The elegant silver and white bottle with the French name came in two sizes. Georgia couldn't resist. She bought the larger one.

A week later while reading the fine print on her elegant (although plastic) bottle, she discovered it contained only one ingredient—water! Georgia had paid $8 for a cup of water! And it wasn't even Perrier.

She felt like a first-class pigeon.

•   •   •

After being taken advantage of or being used, your predominant feeling is anger. Unresolved anger will corrode stomach linings, as well as friendships. Be assured that angry people *always* respond, either outwardly or inwardly.

If you swallow your anger, you have a choice of headaches, ulcers, asthma attacks, back problems, dermatitis, fatigue, insomnia, nerves, and more. Write your own favorite malady here:_____
If you spit your anger out, you may spit on the wrong person. You may be tempted to use others as you have been used.

An amateur manipulator doesn't stand a chance against a professional manipulator. When pigeons use these tactics to retaliate, they often backfire. Pigeons may resort to devious, indirect methods of getting even. Do any of the following sound familiar?

Bitching. Frustrated people do a lot of complaining, griping, backbiting, gossiping, and nagging. Although this is a common response to being used, it is ineffective and more likely to foster tension than relieve it.

Ignoring. When someone asks for help or tries to get you to fetch something, you turn a deaf ear. You try not to acknowledge the other person's presence and may even walk out of the room while he is talking to you.

Sniping. In this form of guerilla warfare, you take potshots at the big shots, hoping to cut them down to size. Sarcasm is a near-lethal weapon if you have a sharp wit and tongue to match. You can be blunt and hurtful in the name of honesty.

Forgetting. "Oops, I forgot." An angry person can easily forget to call Mother, miss committee meetings, fail to keep a doctor's appointment, or leave errands undone.

Procrastinating. A person might agree to cooperate but neglect responsibilities for so long that someone else has to do the task.

Lateness. Being chronically slow or late holds others up, making everyone anxious and irritated. This can also be used by people who want to make a grand entrance.

Sabotage. This is the neat trick of doing work so poorly that you will not be asked to do it again. All it takes is a little carelessness or poor timing.

• • •

Pigeons know these behaviors are childish and petty. (If they don't know, a professional manipulator will be quick to point this out.) After a while, they begin to despise their actions and end up feeling even more foolish, incompetent, and guilty. The net result is a lowered self-esteem, and with a lower self-esteem, the pigeon is even more open to manipulation.

As a woman and a health worker, what are the ploys that have been used against you? Are you more sensitive to approaches through flattery, criticism, insecurity, helplessness, obligation, or guilt? Can you recognize manipulators and manipulation? Can you handle both without feeling angry, bitter, or foolish?

A major goal of assertiveness is to help you discharge anger without going to the extreme of either homicide or suicide. The first step toward resolution is to stop running away. Give yourself permission to be angry. Don't deny and try to hide your true feelings. The next step is to face the person making you miserable. (You may need a mirror to do this.) You have to be willing to look and listen, to acknowledge the other person's presence, along with his or her feelings and opinions. Acknowledgment does not mean agreement.

Who's in charge here?

"Our head nurse was going through a very difficult divorce. She didn't talk about it, but we were all aware of it. The stress began to affect her leadership ability. Since I usually acted as head nurse in her absence, the staff began to turn to me to make decisions and solve problems. This resulted in lots of conflict between me and the head nurse. There was no way to resolve it. I left the job."

Whenever you encounter a situation that everyone knows about but no one is talking about, you are in for trouble. The first step in diffusing the situation is to talk about it.

Sit down with the head nurse. Acknowledge the difficult personal situation she is experiencing. Tell her you know she is going through a rough period, and ask how you can help take the pressure off her at work. If she is vague, you must be specific. List decisions or problems that are waiting for attention. Ask how she would like you to proceed.

If she is still vague, tell her the staff is concerned about her and is hesitant to trouble her at this time. They have asked you for advice and action. Tell her you are uncomfortable being caught in the middle. If you can work through this, conflict will be minimized. It might save your job.

The following is a similar situation in which assertiveness was put to the test:

"I became evening charge nurse, replacing an older nurse who had been demoted after 20 years of service. The staff continued to seek her out to solve problems and make decisions. Finally, I called a meeting of all personnel and told them I was the charge nurse now and I expected to have the problems brought directly to me. Oddly enough, the situation improved tremendously."

It wasn't odd at all. Assertiveness works.

To stop being a pigeon, it is crucial to know what your weaknesses are, because that is where the manipulators will strike first. But a second line of defense is needed in a place where you would least expect it. If the sophisticated manipulators cannot reach you through your weaknesses, they will use your strengths against you.

It has been said that a product's greatest strength is also its greatest weakness. That's a handy thing to remember when a salesman comes knocking at your door. If he praises his product because it is plastic, lightweight, and inexpensive, you can be sure that those advantages are also its disadvantages. You may wish to consider that plastic is nonporous, rigid, tends to crack under pressure, and is difficult to patch or repair. Lightweight? Then it cannot be very substantial or stable. By now, you know that you cannot get something for nothing, so if it is inexpensive, costs had to be cut in materials, labor, or design.

In the same manner, a person's greatest strengths may also be used as weaknesses. Take another look at the list you prepared in Chapter 2. Check your strengths, and think about how they may be used against you:

- Are you a hard worker? Good, then fewer of you have to be hired.
- Are you dedicated? Good, then you can be paid less.
- Are you concerned, caring, and compassionate? Good, then you will find it difficult to ask for a raise or a day off, to refuse to work rotating shifts, overtime, holidays, or weekends.
- Are you dependable? Good, then you won't need much attention.
- Religious? Good, then you know all about giving being better than receiving and turning the other cheek.
- Married? Good, then you don't need a job that can support you, and you will probably get pregnant before you get a promotion or a raise.
- Responsible? Good, then you'll take the blame.

Just as some people are professional manipulators, others are professional pigeons. In the health field alone, there are more than 3 million of us.

Women in the health professions are often taken advantage of in the name of sweet charity. Although salaries for some female health professionals have risen in recent years, in general our salaries can be summed up in three words: cheap, cheap, cheap.

For years we have literally donated our time and talent, believing we were doing so in the service of others. As the injustices and inequities of our health care system become more apparent, some of us are beginning to feel less like angels of mercy and more like accomplices in crime.

Whereas the quality of health care seems to be slipping, the cost of that care is skyrocketing. Coming from middle and lower socioeconomic backgrounds, women health workers know the value of a dollar. We have been highly sensitized to the fact that any increase in our pay, however slight, will be passed along to patients. We have been made to feel guilty for even thinking that we should be financially compensated for our education, work experience, or level of responsibility.

One of the biggest hoaxes ever perpetrated on the American public is that health care is a nonprofit service. Health care is big business. No industry that collects $735 billion a year should be classified as nonprofit. The expenses are huge, but so are the profits. These profits have been siphoned off into the hands of a chosen few: pill producers, building contractors, equipment manufacturers, insurance companies, and physicians. For these people, health care is not a service; it is a bonanza. It is nonprofit only for pigeons and patients.

Health care in the United States can literally be a crime. In Wisconsin, one physician was investigated because it was estimated that he would have had to make a house call every 15 minutes, 7 days a week, 365 days a year, to justify the money he collected from the government through Medicare. It is much safer than sticking up a gas station. Who is going to stick up for us?

Women in the health professions wouldn't mind giving if there weren't so many on the take. Most of us would continue working for peanuts because we honestly care about patients. Money is not the cause of unrest in our ranks. The cause is power. We don't have any.

Many women fear power because of its negative connotations. They picture vindictive, power-mad Amazons whose motto is "Today, the health care industry. Tomorrow, the world!" The power being discussed here is more analogous to electricity: the spark needed to make things move, to get things done. Power to bring energy and light into the health care system. Women have been unplugged too long.

Although men have delegated a lot of responsibility to women, they have not delegated the necessary authority to go with it. If power corrupts and absolute power corrupts absolutely, women are incorruptible. In almost every phase of government, industry, and education, women have no power, no clout.

Check the composition of the Senate and the House of Representatives. Where are the women? Whether you look at industry, politics, academia, or health care, women still account for only about 7 percent of the top officials and administrators.

Women need to regain some of the spunk and spirit they had in the past. For instance, during the late 1800s women owned and operated medical colleges and hospitals of their own because admission to medical schools was denied them. According to Mary Roth Walsh, author of *Doctors Wanted: No Women Need Apply: Sexual Barriers in the Medical Profession 1835-1975,*[*] the turn of the century was a "golden age" for women doctors. In 1900 more than 18 percent of Boston's physicians were women. That figure has not been surpassed to this day. (In 1992 only 17 percent of practicing physicians in the United States were women.)

Eventually, resourcefulness appeared to pay off, and women were granted entrance to the nation's medical schools. By 1894 women represented a significant portion of the student body: as much as 37 percent at Boston University. Believing their battle for sexual equality in medicine had been won, women's rights advocates shifted their attention elsewhere. Convinced that they had outlived their usefulness, 19 separate women's medical colleges closed their doors.

Almost immediately, male physicians declared concern that a surplus of doctors was developing, and they not only reduced enrollments but managed to limit the number of women to 4 or 5 percent of each class. Some fear that a similar backlash against women medical students could develop again today, because although there have been substantial gains, the number of women in influential positions remains unchanged. Medical schools and hospitals have refused to appoint women to key leadership positions. According to the American Medical Association, only 10 percent of medical school faculty members are women, and out of 126 medical schools, only 3 have a woman as dean.

One alternative might be for women to again own and operate institutions themselves. A better alternative might be to make every effort to bypass bureaucracy and institutions altogether.

Muriel Sieh, a social worker in Phoenix, Arizona, is an excellent

---

[*]New Haven, Conn., 1977, Yale University Press.

example of assertiveness in action. A few years ago, her father had been in several unsatisfactory nursing homes. Finally, she found a supportive family that could give him the care he needed. In 3 weeks he began to gain weight, and his monthly medical bills dropped to less than one-fourth their former level.

Convinced she could do this for others as well, she developed the Arizona Adult Foster Home Registry. The foster homes were located through civic and social groups. Depending on the special care needed, boarders were charged from $150 to $600 per month. In the registry's first 2 years of operation, 60 residents found a pleasing alternative to nursing homes or hospitals.

With some imagination and boldness, we might be able to dream up all kinds of alternatives. My favorite health care fantasy is inspired by a mental health institute that charges between $120 and $200 per day. At those rates, the patients should have satin sheets and filet mignon and see Sigmund Freud himself twice a week. Instead, they receive custodial care and are lucky to see a resident who speaks pidgin English once a month. I often think it would be cheaper and more therapeutic to give chronic schizophrenics 90-day passes on Greyhound bus lines and let them stay at Holiday Inn. Don't be afraid to let your imagination run wild. You couldn't possibly dream up any system more outlandish, inefficient, or expensive than the one we already have.

Future trends are bound to take health care out of institutions and back into the home. We cannot afford to do otherwise. When it comes to health care, women are still willing to deliver. Women health workers are already moving out into the community to support families who want to be together during important moments such as when someone is being born or when someone is dying.

Perhaps women should begin to take their business elsewhere. Hit the health industry where it hurts—in the pocketbook. Once we might have been gullible enough to believe that herding people into institutions would result in cheaper, better care. But no more.

If professional women have been pigeons, women patients have been sitting ducks. There is recent and growing evidence that the sexist practices in medicine are hazardous to women's health.

Women's medical complaints still aren't taken seriously. Too often, their symptoms are attributed to stress or emotional disorders.

Myths persist, and they can be deadly. For example, coronary heart disease is seen as a masculine disease, yet it is *the number one killer of women*. Heart disease accounts for half of all women's deaths. Yet even when diagnosed, it is not treated as aggressively in women as in men.

Because their heart disease goes unrecognized for so long, women suffer more complications and a higher mortality rate from heart disease than men.

Even today, there are no clinical studies about how to best treat or prevent heart disease in women. The well-publicized study that promoted taking an aspirin a day to help prevent heart attacks involved over 22,000 *men*. There were no women in the study.

Actually, there are few women in *any* study. We have been excluded because of fear that our hormonal cycles might skew the results. So drugs are tested on men and then fed, by the handfuls, to women. Consider the fact that 75 percent of all mood-altering drugs are consumed by women and yet all the initial trials for antidepressants were done on men. It is shocking!

In 1990 the General Accounting Office released a report criticizing the National Institutes of Health for spending less than 14 percent of its annual budget on research related to women's health. In fact, *only 3 of NIH's 2000 researchers specialized in obstetrics and gynecology.*

Our ignorance is staggering. By making men the norm in clinical trials and definitive research studies, we make women "abnormal." No wonder women's natural biological functions are so often treated like illnesses.

Women continue to be excluded in studies on everything from AIDS to aging. Reproductive health research, a vital concern for women, has been practically abandoned because we have allowed it to become a moral or political issue.

Breast cancer has been a rallying point for many women. In 1989 almost 10 times as much money was allocated for AIDS research at NIH as was allocated for breast cancer research ($750 million as opposed to $77 million). Yet in the past decade women died of breast cancer in numbers as high as almost 10 times the number of people who died of AIDS (430,000 versus 54,000). The numbers don't make sense.

However, there is hope on the horizon. In 1990 Dr. Bernadine Healy became the first women to direct NIH. She announced a separate Women's Health Initiative, funded to the tune of some $600 million and slated to begin in the fall of 1993, which will track diseases such as cancer, heart disease, and osteoporosis in 140,000 women over the next 14 years.

As professionals and as patients, women have been too trusting. We have assumed that men are looking out for our best interests. It appears we have assumed too much.

After several deaths of women on a liquid protein diet were reported, the diet's author was interviewed on national television. It was pointed out to him that all the women had been under medical supervision. His reply was, "There is medical supervision, and then there is medical supervision."

Slowly but surely, women are becoming less gullible, less obedient. We are beginning to be more assertive in seeking health care, in valuing second opinions, in reading and researching illnesses and medications. The first edition of *Our Bodies, Ourselves** was a landmark in helping us understand our bodies enough to seek informed medical care.

Seeking medical care and seeking health care are two entirely different things. Unfortunately, the terms are so often used interchangeably that they are assumed to be synonymous. But medical care is care given by physicians, whereas health care encompasses the valuable services rendered by dietitians, psychologists, pharmacists, · dentists, nurses, physical therapists, and others in addition to doctors.

When the term "physician extender" was introduced, all I could think of was grinding up soybeans to make sirloin go farther. Personally, I don't enjoy being thought of as the soy of life. Although I wouldn't object to being called a "health care extender," I find "physician extender" offensive. Now some hospitals are hiring "nurse extenders" to work with nurses.

Many doctors are very good at what they do, but what they do is more limited than anyone is willing to admit. It is estimated that 75 percent of all symptoms are not related to any organic disease but to tension, depression, frustration, loneliness, lack of coping skills, poor interpersonal relationships, and so forth. No amount of surgery or drugs can correct these problems. However, read *JAMA*, and you will find its content almost exclusively related to organic disease. Doctors concentrate on tissue damage, not on damage to the individual or the family.

Furthermore, it is estimated that 20 percent of all patients in a typical research hospital acquire an iatrogenic disease. *Iatrogenic.* Sounds like a new virus, but it means "physician-induced." Translated, that means that 20 percent of patients have to be treated for problems resulting from medical treatment itself.

---

*Boston Women's Health Book Collective, New York, 1973, Simon & Schuster.

Finally, women are beginning to question whether the team concept is viable in our present system. Our health care system has never been a democracy. It is a dictatorship. It might best be compared with a game in which the child who owns the ball refuses to play unless the others agree to play by his or her rules and his or her rules alone. Under such circumstances, even if a team is organized, it can never be a winning one.

Perhaps it was a mistake to admit women to institutions of higher learning. The more we learn, the less we understand. We do not understand why our salaries, fringe benefits, and advancement opportunities should be less than those of men. Even more important, we do not understand why we are allowed no voice and no vote in the policies and practices of the health care industry. We pigeons have toed the line long enough.

In closing this chapter, let us all stand and sing the rousing "Battle Hymn of Uppity Nurses."

BATTLE HYMN OF UPPITY NURSES

Words: Melodie Chenevert
Music: Slightly borrowed.*

I joined the health professions
To fight pain and misery
But after my 8 hours
I'm the one in agony
So much to do, so little time
It really is a shame—
And I'm the one they blame

Chorus
Don't let the health industry
   screw ya
Get what you've got coming to ya
The quality of care will soon
   unglue ya
If the patient's just a pawn

I worked on Christmas, New Year's
Thanksgiving and Halloween
I'm not sure but I think I had
A weekend in between
Rotating shifts and lack of help
Can make a person mean—
When the patient's just a pawn

Reporting off I wished the next shift
"Bon voyage, good luck!"
We've 17 on critical
And 12 IV's are stuck
The resident is deaf and dumb
The laundry's gone amuck—
And the patient's just a pawn

I work hard as any surgeon
But I rarely hear a "thanks"
I'm still saving for support hose
He's got money in Swiss banks
If you think that this is quite unfair
Then come and join our ranks—
Or the patient's just a pawn

---

*To be sung to the tune of "Battle Hymn of the Republic," sometimes better known as "Glory, Glory, Hallelujah." Should be accompanied by kazoos or the local philharmonic—whichever is cheaper.

10

What's good for the goose . . .

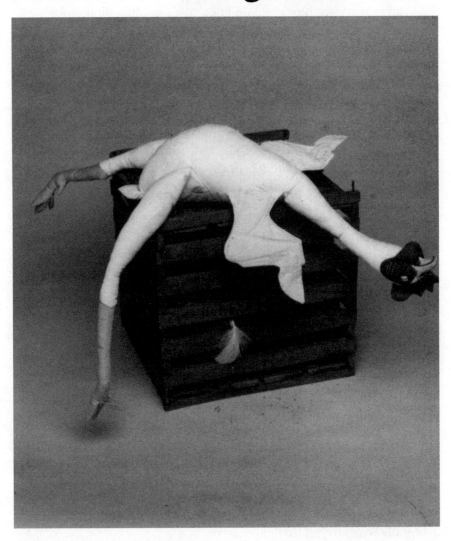

Birds of a feather.

hat's good for the goose? A job. Preferably one with significant status and salary. Women who work outside the home are healthier and happier (even though they are more harried) than those who do not. However, although combining marriage, motherhood, and a successful career may be a good idea, it is one that is exceedingly difficult to implement. Any of you who have struggled with a dual-career marriage plus children know just how difficult it is.

By choosing one of the health professions, you may have thought a career would automatically follow. But entering a profession is one thing, and building a career is quite another.

A career is more than a series of jobs. It is a demanding commitment that requires investment and sacrifice. In return, a career pays off handsomely in tangible and intangible ways. The more responsibility assumed, the greater the reward and recognition. Status and salary spiral upward.

Unfortunately, many women in the health professions have discovered that their career path is not leading upward. While there is no limit to the amount of responsibility they are expected to assume, there is often very limited potential for reward or recognition.

Harold Geneen, writing in *Managing,* says that workers are paid in two coins: one is money, and the other is experience. He says if you get the experience, the money will follow. That may be true for men, but there is little evidence it holds true for women. Salaries for most women in the health professions are "compressed," meaning there is little difference in earning power between the experienced and the inexperienced.

Women's career ladders seem to be more horizontal than vertical. The next rung of the ladder isn't up; it is just one notch to the left or the right of our present position.

For example, Fran was recently offered a position with a state agency. The title was impressive, but the salary was not, and there was no room to negotiate, since the salary was set by the legislature. The recruiter, eager to convince Fran to sign on, assured her that "the experience would be invaluable."

Fran smiled and declined, saying she had taken other nursing jobs that promised a wealth of experience but had found there was no way to literally "cash in" on that experience.

Instead of criticizing women for lack of career commitment, perhaps we should take a closer look at how much a career actually delivers to a woman in return for her investment and sacrifice. Why should women put career first unless the relationship is reciprocal?

As the number of dual-career couples grows, so do the problems associated with maintaining intimate relationships while tending to business.

> Heather is a dentist, and her husband, Rob, is a physician. Three years ago they moved from an apartment into their dream home. Soon after, the nightmares began. Neither realized how much time and energy it takes to clean, repair, and maintain your own property.
>
> Both had growing practices with long hours and unpredictable schedules. They barely saw each other during the week, and when the weekend came, they spent it doing "homework." Heather cleaned, laundered, shopped, and ran errands. Rob mowed, weeded, serviced the cars, and did home repairs.
>
> Their social life was nil. Being together was no fun, because they were either doing chores or arguing about who was supposed to do the chores. Both were tired and irritable. Fearing their marriage was collapsing, they sought counseling. The counselor agreed they needed help—the domestic kind. His prescription? Hire a housekeeper. Having a housekeeper made such a dramatic difference that a month later they also hired a gardener. Yes, it is expensive, but Heather and Rob say it is a lot cheaper than psychotherapy or divorce.

Dual-career couples require outside help. If your "job" enables you to employ substantial household help, you probably have a career. If your "career" does not enable you to use such services, you probably only have a job.

Actually, the number of dual-career couples is relatively small. A more accurate term for most of us would be "double-income couples," because there is usually a primary and a secondary wage earner. Guess who has subordinate status. The wife. Frankly, few wives can afford careers, because for all practical purposes women still have total responsibility for child care and household chores.

Before women can fully invest in careers, two issues must be resolved: housework and child care.

Housework

When conducting workshops on goal setting, I ask women to fill in this blank: "One thing I want that would make my personal/professional life more satisfying is _____." I let participants brainstorm and generate a group wish list.

Invariably, HOUSEKEEPER is mentioned and draws applause. Other people listed often include a nanny, maid, cook, chauffeur, and secretary. These people represent services that women frequently provide for their husbands but husbands rarely, if ever, provide for their wives. Career women often express the need for a "wife"—that person who performs a myriad of tasks like shopping, cooking, cleaning, tending, mending, delivering, typing, finding, and fetching. And all without costing a dime!

Recently it was suggested that wives of diplomats should be salaried because they provide so many services and are expected to make so many sacrifices for their husbands' careers. That notion was quickly quieted.

While today's women are expected to bring home the bacon, today's men are still not expected to fry it. Almost every working woman must moonlight as a housewife, but almost no working man moonlights as a househusband.

> "On my third 12-hour night shift, I got up at 4 PM to get ready for work at 7:30. My husband was watching TV. I took a shower and asked him what was for dinner. He said, 'I don't know—leftovers?' I said, 'Well, get them ready.'
>
> We ate, and suddenly I was crying and saying all kinds of things to him like: Why can't he make dinner for me when I'm working? I make dinner for him when I'm off. Why do I have to remind him? We have to eat! Would I send him to work without dinner? Of course not! What a double standard!"

Another crying jag for a woman on stress overload. Another woman with a rigorous, exhausting professional life who receives little or no support around the house.

> "I worked a 12-hour shift and came home to find unexpected company. I prepared supper and entertained them until after midnight.
>
> When I came home from work the next night, my husband informed me the place was a *mess*. I sat down on the couch, closed my eyes, and said, 'He who sees it, cleans it.'
>
> After the initial shock, my husband burst out laughing. He helped me clean up the mess but let me know it was *my* responsibility and he was doing me a *favor* by helping."

Few men seem to have gotten the message about how couples are supposed to be sharing the scut work that goes with maintaining hearth and home.

> "After working a full 8-hour shift at the hospital and another 5 or 6 hours as a secretary for my husband's business, I came home and cooked supper.

Just as I was ready to go to bed, my husband said, 'I have no clean underwear for my trip tomorrow.'"

This is an excellent situation to role-play. It hits a raw nerve for most working women and lends itself beautifully to a variety of passive, aggressive, and assertive responses.

For example, you might passively trudge down to the basement, fuming all the way, and toss in a load of clothes. You might aggressively scream at him that you are not an indentured servant and that he can jolly well wash his own clothes. You might assertively say, "You do have a problem. What are you going to do about it?"

When one of my colleagues had a similar experience, she said to her husband, "Oh, don't you know you can just turn your underwear inside out? And they're good for another 3 days!" Then she went to bed.

Studies continue to show that even husbands who are unemployed do much less housework than their wives who are employed full-time. Even well-educated couples who profess to believe in full sharing of household tasks and child-rearing responsibilities, rarely practice what they preach. Evidently men's aversion to housework is so intense that domestic chores can become a battleground on which more than one marriage has been crippled or killed.

Neither men nor women value housework. The assumption is: any village idiot can do it. Not true.

I have a lot of talents. Housekeeping is just not among them. Having sons, a German shepherd, and a husband with no more talent for or interest in domestic chores than I do, the house is usually a disaster. I try to keep the clutter from posing a serious health hazard. It's a thankless job, but someone has to do it. When clutter and chaos overwhelm me, I have a hysterical outburst that temporarily mobilizes every family member. They pitch in and help with the tiresome chores.

Every now and then, I get desperate enough to consider hiring outside help. One day several years ago when I was especially vulnerable, I noticed a neatly printed sign on the grocery store bulletin board saying "Marie" was anxious to find housekeeping jobs. And she was cheap! I called the number listed, and an hour later the doorbell rang.

When I opened the door, I found a dumpy, disheveled young woman with dark hair awry and teeth protruding in several directions. I took one look at her and said to myself, "No one is going to hire this woman." So I hired her.

It turned out Marie was no better at housework than I was. So I rolled up my sleeves and worked alongside her.

Marie had dropped out of high school a couple of years earlier. She hoped to be married soon, but there was a slight hitch. Her boyfriend might have to go to jail. He had been arrested three times for petty theft and was due to face the judge for sentencing in several weeks. If he got off (again) with probation, they would be married. If he had to go to jail, the wedding would be postponed.

As I worked with Marie, I did my best psychiatric nurse impression. I listened, I probed, I counseled, and I cleaned house. I loaned her money to enter a tutoring program so she could get her high school equivalency diploma.

Poor Marie had no aptitude for housework. She gave everything a lick and a promise, then dashed off.

After noticing one of Marie's particularly sloppy jobs, my husband turned to me and said, "Mel, this just isn't working out. You're going to have to fire her."

"I can't fire her," I moaned.

"What do you mean you can't fire her? You wrote the book on assertiveness!"

"I can't fire her. If I fire her, she'll get married, and then there will be 12 offspring with hair awry and protruding teeth ringing my doorbell and looking for work. And I'll feel responsible and have to hire them all!"

Marie continued to work for me another month. Then one day she came and announced she had to quit. I resisted the urge to shout a joyful "Thank God!" and asked her what was happening.

Marie reminded me she was scheduled to take her high school equivalency exam the following week. She told me she had finally broken up with her boyfriend and added, "You know, if I'm ever going to make anything of myself, I have to have a full-time job. I went to the state employment agency, and they found a job for me. The bad part is I can't work for you anymore."

I congratulated her, wished her well, sent her on her way, and locked the door behind her.

My house is still a total disaster. But every time I think about hiring help, a picture of Marie pops into my mind. Then I roll up my sleeves and do it myself.

Like so many other women in the health professions, I try to be "therapeutic" to everyone. I am a sucker for hard-luck stories. I feel duty bound to help people at home, at work, at play. It's exhausting.

To survive in a dual-career marriage, charity must not only begin at home, it must end at home. You and I have to learn to curb our rescue-mission impulses when hiring or firing. We have to make sure that hired help is really *hired help* and not just an extension of our caseload.

We also have to get over our hang-up on housework being woman's work. We have to stop feeling ashamed when we hire a housekeeper.

> "I have had a cleaning lady for 3 years. Many of my friends and family don't know this. I am too ashamed."

We need to approach housework in a more intelligent manner. Here's a woman who did:

> "My husband and I both work full-time. (We have no children.) For years I took responsibility for *all* of the housework, cooking, shopping, errands, etc. Finally, I woke up. I insisted we start sharing the chores.
>
> This lead to many heated discussions. Then only rarely and reluctantly would my husband help with vacuuming or doing the dishes. I was becoming very angry at the unfairness of all of this.
>
> Finally, I decided if he wouldn't do any of the housework, neither would I. I hired a housekeeper. It is great! I wish I had done it *years* ago!"

Child care

My sister and her husband are *dinks,* a marketing acronym that stands for "double income, no kids." Like many dual-career couples they literally can't conceive of complicating their lives further by having children. However, *90 percent* of all American women will conceive and complicate their lives, not to mention their careers, by having children.

Unlike my sister, I have struggled to have it all—marriage, career, and children. The operative word is struggled. Striving to be successful in all three areas is a spectacular juggling act bordering on the impossible. While some of us make it look easy, it never is.

When a colleague gave birth to twins at age 40, it sparked a round-table discussion about the joys and tribulations of motherhood. All of us were professional women in our late thirties and early forties with older school-age or teenage children. One co-worker said she thought having a "change of life" baby would keep her young. In contrast, I was sure having a baby at my age would take years off my life. It would kill me to have to go through the agony of making child care arrangements again.

For many of us, the most difficult part of having it all is finding adequate child care. Very few employers provide subsidies or facilities for child care. Of mothers with children under 1 year of age, over half now hold jobs. This is very troubling, because while child care is in short supply at every age, it is particularly scarce for infants. Affluence doesn't count. Good child care may not be available at any price.

Even *married* working women often feel like single parents. Mothers are the ones who must scramble to piece together a crazy patchwork of babysitting arrangements. Mothers are the ones who stay home with a sick child. Mothers are the ones who compromise their careers and adjust their schedules for as much at-home time as possible. Mothers are the ones who are wracked with guilt.

Women continue to accept minor roles in the workplace because they must continue to play the major role on the home front. The lack of adequate child care often keeps women in part-time jobs with little career mobility. It restricts women to jobs for which they are overqualified and prevents them from accepting or seeking promotions.

The epitomy of this crisis? When Zoe Baird was nominated for Attorney General of the United States in early 1993 and had to withdraw because of hiring an illegal alien to provide child care. It was called a scandal. What was, and still is, scandalous is the appalling lack of competent child care available to rich and poor alike.

Accepting and seeking promotions can be a watershed for dual-career couples. If a man is offered a promotion that involves a geographic change, he will accept and "hope" his wife will be able to resume her career in the new locale. If a wife is offered a promotion that involves a move, she will decline unless her husband can be properly relocated and his career does not suffer in the transition. Perhaps that is one reason professional women continue to make only two thirds of what their male counterparts earn.

After living a few years in a community that offered me no career opportunities, I accepted the challenge of setting up a nursing program 300 miles from home. It meant leaving my husband and sons to fend for themselves. And it meant I had to fend for myself for the first time in years.

I worked on the project for 3 months and then returned home for the summer. Knowing I would have to finish the project in the fall, our sons (ages 10 and 14) chose to go with me and spend the school year on the Oregon coast. The experience was exhilarating, exasperating, and exhausting. While our marriage probably became stronger during this period, my husband and I agreed that long-distance parenting is impractical at best. The boys and I returned to home base.

A year after I had finished that project, I was offered a wonderful position *only* 200 miles from home. I could not accept. I felt I had other promises to keep. Unspoken promises made when our sons were born.

The cost of *pursuing* a career is just too high for most wives and mothers. So if you are a dual-career couple, choose your community carefully. Make sure there are more than jobs available. Make sure there are career opportunities for both of you.

While over 100 nations provide maternity or parental leave as a matter of national policy, the United States did not until January 1993. Most of those countries also make child care a national priority, providing facilities and subsidies. The United States does not. For years we have known that our infant mortality rate is shameful compared with many other industrialized countries. Evidently our lack of commitment to child care is just as shameful. We say the United States is child-centered, but our actions (or lack of actions) contradict our words.

In this country child care has been seen as a private, individual problem and more specifically as a woman's problem. Until now, our government has seemed oblivious to the needs of working women and their children. Perhaps that is not surprising when you realize the House and Senate are made up almost exclusively of men, predominantly from law and business, of whom 70 percent are reported millionaires. What is surprising is that women's advocacy and feminist groups seem to be almost as oblivious to these needs.

In our haste to secure *equal* treatment for women, we have ignored the fact that women carry an *unequaled* responsibility for the preservation and continuation of society.

It is true, only women can have babies; it is both the privilege and the responsibility of the female sex. To ignore this biological difference, as many American feminists chose to do, is to commit a double folly. In the first place, it ensures that most women will become second-class citizens in the workplace. *For without public support policies few women can cope with motherhood without hopelessly compromising their career goals.* Secondly, society has to suffer. For a child cannot be compared with a new car or a vacation, some private consumer good that a woman can choose to spend resources on if the fancy strikes her. The decision to have a child is both a private and a public decision, for children are our collective future.*

Abortion steals the spotlight, and no one seems to care a feather or a fig about children once they are born. Since 1980 federal policies and slashed appropriations have catapulted alarming numbers of children into poverty. Democratic Representative Barney Frank from Massachusetts once quipped that Ronald Reagan seemed to believe "life begins at conception and ends at birth." Now it is Bill Clinton's turn to lead the country. Let's see if his promises and policies are more child-friendly.

When it comes to child-care issues, our behavior to date has been passive-aggressive. On the passive side, we ignore the changes in our society that have made child care crucial. Denying there is a problem, we do little or nothing. On the aggressive side, we shame and blame working mothers. We look for scapegoats, not solutions.

Today we need assertive action: bold, confident, positive. For example, one approach that might prove beneficial to both dual-career couples and their children would be to expand the school day and the school year. Our school year is 25 percent shorter than that of other advanced countries. In England, for instance, children attend school 8 hours a day, 220 days a year, while here in the United States children attend school 6 hours a day, 180 days a year. By increasing the time our children spend in school, we might not only improve their academic abilities, but also take some pressure off working parents to provide child care.

For child care, unlike housework, is not *your* problem or *my* problem. It is *our* problem. Correction—it is our OPPORTUNITY to shape the future.

As women in the health professions, we are fully aware of the foundations of good mental and physical health. Shouldn't we be in the vanguard championing the cause of child care? It doesn't matter if your children have already left the nest or if you're a "dink"; let's begin to work together for the future.

What's good for the goose is good for the gander . . . and for the goslings.

---

*From Hewlett, Sylvia Ann: *A Lesser Life,* New York, 1986, Warner Books, p. 147.

11

Nest eggs

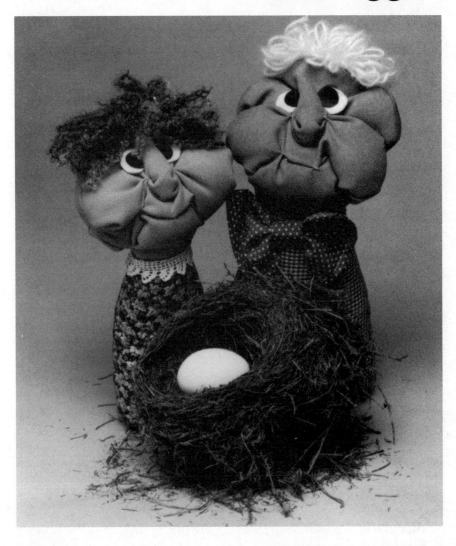

Nest eggs.

As a young couple with a growing family, we decided we should have our insurance policies reviewed and updated. We invited the company representative to our home. As soon as we sat down at the dining room table, he launched into a tragic scenario aimed at me.

"What would you do if Gary died tomorrow?" he demanded dramatically.

"First I'd cry, and then I'd bury him," I replied with a half smile.

"But what would you do if he died, the furnace blew up, and there was no milk in the refrigerator?"

"I'd cry, bury him, call the repairman, and go to the grocery store," I giggled. His melodramatic tactics were wasted on us.

We couldn't be frightened into buying more insurance. We told him we would be uncomfortable knowing we were worth more dead than alive, and since we had both invested heavily in education, we had the best possible form of insurance.

"But what about disability? What about retirement?" He made a last attempt to persuade us to insure ourselves to the hilt.

We were betting we wouldn't be disabled. And retirement? Frankly, it is difficult to think about, let alone prepare for retirement when you've barely launched your career.

When it became obvious that he was not going to be able to sell us more insurance, he switched products and began telling us about the company's newly formed mutual fund. That caught our attention. We invested $1000 and essentially forgot about it.

Over 10 years passed before we had our insurance reviewed again. Although we were sitting around a new dining room table, in a new house, in a new state, with a new salesman, it was the old husband-dies-furnace-blows-no-milk scenario all over again. While the scare tactics were no more effective this time than last time, something did jolt us out of our complacency. The fact that we were 10 years older and were not much sounder financially than we had been when we first began our careers startled us. We immediately opened Individual Retirement Accounts, diverted money into that mutual fund before it reached our checking account, and began a small but consistent savings plan.

An episode at a workshop I was conducting brought these memories to mind. In the past couple of years I have done a lot of work with women health professionals related to setting goals and establishing priorities. Generally, I have found that women have few goals but many dreams. (The difference between a dream and a goal is a workable plan.) When it comes to money management, many women have wild fantasies instead of goals.

Women are very aware of the "biological clock" that limits the number of childbearing years. Yet women seem totally unaware of the "financial clock" that is simultaneously ticking away.

One of my favorite cartoons shows an anguished career woman with head in hands groaning, "I can't believe I forgot to have children." Just as there are time limits on filling your nest, there are time limits on feathering your nest. Don't be caught groaning, "I can't believe I forgot to make retirement plans."

Several years ago while addressing a nursing convention, I suggested we all become actively involved in recruiting nursing students for purely selfish reasons. Calling attention to participants with "a few silver hairs among the gold," I told them the severe drop in enrollment in 1985, 1986, and 1987 coupled with the increased demand for nurses meant an impending shortage so severe nurses might never be allowed to retire. There would simply be no one to replace them. When I pantomimed a nurse hobbling around in a walker still dispensing medications, everyone roared with laughter.

During the break period, a nurse in her early sixties approached me. "Just tell me how I am going to retire even if there are younger nurses to replace me! I can't afford to retire—THERE'S NO MONEY!" For her, this was no laughing matter. She was frantic.

Like so many other women, she had spent a lifetime caring for others while giving little thought to her own care. Although she may have made every day count, she had nothing to count on for tomorrow. And she is not alone. Her lack of financial planning is not the exception; it's the rule.

A Princeton University study commissioned by Merrill Lynch & Co. and released in January 1993 suggests that only 10 to 20 percent of us are saving enough money to retire in comfort. Put another way, 80 to 90 percent of us will not be spending our "golden" years in comfort.

The problem is directly linked to our poor savings record. The average U.S. citizen saves less than 5 percent a year, whereas the average Japanese citizen saves over 20 percent.

Here's more good financial news for women. Because we earn less and live longer than men, it is recommended that we begin saving at an earlier age and squirreling away a higher percentage of our meager income. A double whammy!

Most women also need to prepare for another eventuality—widowhood. An excellent book has become available: *On Your Own: A Widow's Passage to Emotional & Financial Well-Being*. Authors Alexandra Armstrong, a nationally known certified financial planner, and Mary R. Donahue, a psychologist, have teamed up to cover everything you need to know to successfully navigate this difficult transition. Their book is unique because it combines information on how to cope with the emotional and financial turmoil widowhood brings. Neither issue can be overlooked if the woman is to regain a sense of security and well-being.

The authors are compassionate, intelligent, and extremely practical. There are checklists and worksheets along with down-to-earth suggestions for dealing with agencies and advisors. They guide you through the immediate crisis and help you build a secure future. Information covered includes such things as calculating your net worth, protecting your assets, basic rules of investing, and establishing your new identity.

For many of us "financial planning" means making the money last through the month. We tend to live to the limits of our income. As our salaries increase, so does our spending. We pay off the house, we pay off the car, we pay off the doctor, we pay off all the bills. We pay off everyone but ourselves.

According to financial experts, however, the key to building a nest egg is to pay yourself—FIRST! Before you write out a check to the gas company or the orthodontist, write out a check to yourself. You sock away a percentage of your income consistently every month. One of the easiest ways is to have an automatic payroll deduction that transfers a specific amount to a savings account so that a portion of your paycheck never reaches the checking account. Because, once money reaches the checking account, it's as good as gone. The out-of-sight-out-of-mind principle works for most women, and the savings begin to grow.

If you want to accumulate $100,000 by age 65, how much would you have to put away each month? Based on 5 percent interest compounded annually, if you began saving at age 35 it would take $119 per month; at age 45 it would take $240.50 per month; and at age 55 it would take $632 per month. There are two messages here: start young and put your money where it will earn a lot more than 5 percent.

Venita Van Caspel, author of *The Power of Money Dynamics,* suggests a *$300,000* nest egg if you want to achieve financial independence. Her book is an excellent guide to converting your financial fantasies into achievable goals.

You may approach financial planning passively, assertively, or aggressively. Unfortunately, the passive approach is most common.

Financially passive

If you are financially passive, you don't plan. You assume. You assume someone else, whether it is your spouse or the Social Security system, will take care of money matters.

Afraid to look foolish, you keep silent. You don't ask questions. You consider discussions of money unladylike.

The financial page of the newspaper looks like gibberish, so you turn it over and clip the coupons on the back, not realizing you are the one getting clipped. Saving 25 cents on cereal is ludicrous when hundreds and thousands of dollars are slipping away. Ignorance is expensive.

You procrastinate. Worried about making a wrong decision on financial matters, you make no decision. You keep waiting for the "right" time to begin saving or investing. There is only one right time—NOW.

You and your husband never discuss how you will manage financially after his death, even though statistics say you will outlive him an average of 7 years (assuming you are the same age). Not only will you be grief-stricken after his death, you will be poverty-stricken.

As you move in and out of the workplace to follow your husband or tend your children, you never calculate the cost of lost pension benefits. You accept part-time or dead-end jobs that offer no benefits. The Older Women's League (OWL) says that only 2 out of 10 women receive any pension benefits based on either their own or their husband's earnings.

You close your eyes, cross your fingers, and buy lottery tickets. You end up a near–bag lady, too soon old and too late smart. Perhaps this grim picture will spur you into positive action.

Financially assertive

If you want to be financially assertive, you will stop assuming and start planning. You will not expect someone else to look out for your financial future. You will take charge.

You will read, study, question, calculate, evaluate, and take action. You will identify short-term and long-term financial goals and develop workable plans to achieve them. Realizing that it is not how much money you make over your lifetime that counts, but how much you manage to keep, you will hire an accountant and a financial planner.

You will develop a positive attitude about money—both making it and managing it. There are lots of publications available, such as *Business Week, Business Woman, Inc., Money, Venture, Forbes,* and the *Wall Street Journal.* They are recreational reading compared with the professional journals you wade through each month. If you are tired of reading, there is a videotape produced by *Forbes* called *The Joy of Stocks.* Look for it the next time you rent a movie video. In the same time it would take to watch Clint Eastwood in *A Fistful of Dollars,* you can learn essential financial management information that will help you make a fistful of your own.

Because you are financially assertive, you will know your net worth. If you haven't done that calculation lately, do it now.

Assets

House (current market value)	_____
Car (current market value)	_____
Money in checking account	_____
Money in savings account	_____
Stocks, bonds	_____
Personal property (furniture, jewelry, antiques)	_____
Cash value of insurance policies	_____
Other	_____
TOTAL	$_____

Liabilities

Mortgages	_____
Installment loans	_____
Credit card debts	_____
Taxes	_____
Other	_____
TOTAL	$_____

$$\begin{array}{r}\text{Assets}\\ -\text{ Liabilities}\\ \hline \text{Net worth}\end{array}$$

Whether your net worth is impressive or depressive, you will budget—not with a sense of aggravation but with a sense of anticipation. Someone quipped, "Savings is just delayed spending." Take a good look at your monthly income and your monthly outgo. Fill in the appropriate spaces for the last 12 months. See the form on pp. 144-145.

Take a moment to compare your actual spending habits with those recommended. First, fill in the blank: "My actual take-home pay each month is $_____." Now fill in the boxes based on that figure and contrast it with your own income/outgo figures from the previous exercise.

	Recommended Amount	Amount I Spent
Recommended Distribution of Total Income (%)	$_____	$_____
House 25%-30%	_____	_____
Food 12%-14%	_____	_____
Insurance 5%-7%	_____	_____
Transportation 5%-7%	_____	_____
Recreation 4%-6%	_____	_____
Clothing 6%-7%	_____	_____
Savings/investments 5%-25%	_____	_____

You will begin a consistent savings plan to establish a READY fund. That way, if any emergencies or opportunities arise, you will be ready. Financial advisors recommend you keep 4 to 6 month's income readily accessible. Accessible does not mean tucked under the mattress but deposited in a savings account or a money fund that allows you quick access without penalty.

You will make sure your insurance protection is adequate but not excessive. Before making any insurance decisions, be sure to study Van Caspel's book.

Once you have analyzed your assets, formulated financial plans, established a "ready" fund, and protected yourself with adequate insurance, you are ready to begin investing in something like the Individual Retirement Account (IRA) or Simplified Employee Pension Plan (SEP). These are highly recommended because they provide substantial tax benefits.

For example, if you invest $2000 in an IRA at 10 percent annual interest, in 10 years you will have $5200. If you place that same $2000 in a savings account paying 10 percent annual interest and you are in a 33 percent tax bracket, in 10 years it will be worth $2500.

When you finally have all these financial ducks in a row, you can invest in the stock market. Whether you choose stocks or bonds or a combination of both, think safety first. Look for steady growth over the

Income	Jan	Feb	Mar	Apr	May
Salary					
Dividends					
Interest					
Capital gains					
Other					

Expenses					
Rent/mortgage					
Food					
Utilities					
Transportation					
Taxes					
Health care					
Child care					
Education					
Clothing					
Personal stuff					
Entertainment					
Insurance					
Savings					
Investments					
Other					

June	July	Aug	Sep	Oct	Nov	Dec

long haul—sort of a get-rich-slow approach. You will need expert advice because most of us are too busy making money to do an optimum job of managing the money we make.

Financially aggressive

If you are financially aggressive, it could mean you use money to control, threaten, or injure others, but it merely means you take a lot more risks than others do. Instead of investing for safe, long-term growth, you play the stock market. You move your money about quickly. You gamble on high-return or no-return propositions.

If you are wise, you invest only a tiny portion of your assets this way. Get-rich-quick dreams frequently turn into nightmares. Never invest money this way that you are not prepared to lose.

If you want to learn more about taking charge of your financial future, see the annotated bibliography at the end of this book. It is not the information but the way you use this information that will determine whether you end your career with a large nest egg or a large goose egg.

12

From barnyard to mountaintop

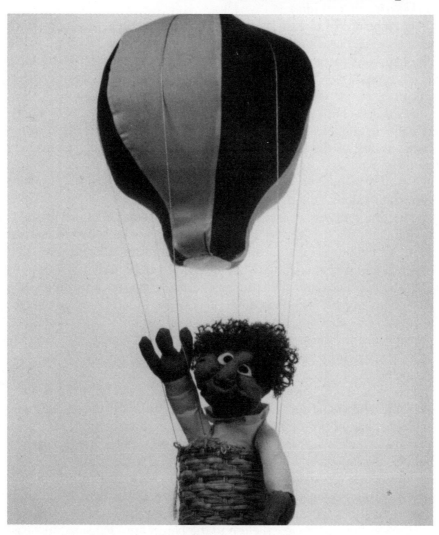

*It takes more than hot air
to make dreams come true.*

The Colorado Nurses' Association once called to see if I could give a workshop on "advanced assertiveness." Being very bold, confident, and positive, I assured them I could. Frankly, at that moment I didn't know what advanced assertiveness was, but if I couldn't find it, I would invent it. (Some shameless people will do anything to get out of the barnyard and up to mountaintops as beautiful as those in Vail, Colorado.)

Even before I hung up the phone, I was mentally trying to differentiate between basic and advanced assertiveness. While I worked on the problem, four categories or levels of assertiveness began to take shape. They crystallized into remedial assertiveness, basic assertiveness, advanced assertiveness, and beyond assertiveness (Table 1).

Remedial assertiveness. Table 1 can be read both vertically and horizontally. To help clarify the material condensed there, let's begin with a verbal sketch of the woman who is in need of remedial assertiveness training. First and foremost, she has little or no self-esteem. Feeling inadequate in most of life's arenas, she frequently belittles her ability, education, talent, and experience.

Her prime directive is to avoid conflict at all costs. That's why she is so reluctant to use the word "no." Saying no to someone causes conflict. Quiet, obedient, and conforming, she allows and even depends on others to tell her what to do and where to go.

Although there are many things she really doesn't want to do, she does them anyway. "If I don't do it, no one else will," she sighs. It never occurs to her that if she is the *only* person willing to do something, perhaps it is not worth doing.

A martyr in the making, she tends to be self-sacrificing and masochistic. She tries to use guilt to control others, even as she is controlled by it. Having resigned herself to making do with whatever is available, she would not presume to ask for what she needs, let alone what she wants. Seeing herself as a victim of fate (culture, sex, time, space) she feels powerless to make changes in her life. She has dreams but few aspirations and no goals.

She is a nice person, a polite person. She is also fearful, depressed, and very tired. Blinded by anxiety, she sees no alternatives. She simply does what she is told and wishes everyone else would do the same.

To help her venture even close to the borderline that separates passive from assertive behavior will require weeks, months, or perhaps years of gentle coaching and systematic, sympathetic support.

Basic assertiveness. Contrast the woman at the remedial assertive-

Table 1 Four levels of assertiveness

Remedial Assertiveness	Basic Assertiveness	Advanced Assertiveness	Beyond Assertiveness
Low self-esteem	Budding self-esteem	High self-esteem plus . . .	. . . High esteem for others
Afraid to say no	Delights in saying no	Comfortable saying no	BUT delights in saying yes
Masochistic	**Sadistic**		**Holistic**
Avoids conflict at all costs	Handles uncomplicated conflict comfortably	Recognizes conflict as potentially positive; enjoys seeking resolution	Willing to take risks personally and professionally
Anxiety	**Action**	**Energy**	**Power**
Knows what she doesn't want but does it anyway	Knows what she doesn't want and refuses to do it	Knows what she wants and . . .	. . . Is not afraid to go for it!
Dependent	**Obstinate**	**Independent**	**Interdependent**
Sees no alternatives	Is aware alternatives exist	Chooses from alternatives	Invents alternatives
Hides	Seeks	Self-directed	Sought by others
External locus of control		**Internal locus of control**	
Hourly/daily planning	Monthly/yearly planning	3-, 5-, 10-year planning	Planning for a lifetime and beyond
Lets others define goals	Defines own goals	Has definite goals and workable plans for achieving them	Continually formulates, updates, redefines, and prioritizes goals
Considers own time, talent, education, and experience inadequate	Begins to value own time, talent, education, and experience	High regard for own time, talent, education, and experience	Values time, talent, education, and experience of others

ness stage with the one who has achieved a basic assertiveness level in theory and practice. Here is a woman who has begun to value her time, talent, education, and experience. Her budding self-esteem is fragile but growing stronger each day.

Handling uncomplicated conflicts with waiters, clerks, mechanics, and virtual strangers is a snap. She has even been known to confront some people in high places like her boss, minister, and husband. Busy testing old relationships, values, and stereotypes, she enjoys flexing her newfound mental, physical, and emotional muscles.

Suddenly aware that alternatives exist, she begins weighing choices, making changes, and taking chances. She devotes time and energy to plans and activities that will enhance *her* personal and professional life.

In many ways it is a selfish time. After years of passive, cooperative behavior in which she has ignored her own needs and catered to the wants and wishes of others, she begins putting herself first. When asked to do chores and tasks that she doesn't want to do, she refuses. She refuses with almost sadistic glee.

For the woman at this level, assertiveness is more likely to be used as a weapon than a tool. Her attitude and behavior changes often confuse and alienate those around her. Although she is not as easily affected by guilt, she is not immune to it, either.

This rather negative but necessary phase is disruptive and uncomfortable. So uncomfortable that the weak may retreat and return to passiveness . . . and Valium. Others, too aware to return to old attitudes and behaviors, yet too fearful or shortsighted to push ahead, accept the elementary gains of basic assertiveness. They are content with what they have learned in Assertiveness 101. However, the strong and those blessed with support and encouragement continue exploring, exercising, and experimenting with assertiveness. They are the ones who will go on to advanced assertiveness.

Advanced assertiveness. To reach this third level of assertiveness, a woman must outgrow the depression of the first level and the anger of the second. She has to make the critical connection between assertiveness and achievement.

The woman who masters advanced assertiveness has high regard for her own time, talent, education, and experience. Not only does she have definite personal and professional goals, she also has workable plans for achieving them. Having assimilated assertiveness, she uses it skillfully to save time and energy and to move forward toward her goals. She is a woman who knows what she wants and is no longer afraid to go after it.

Unlike a woman at a lower level of assertiveness who floats adrift at the mercy of people, places, and events (external locus of control), the woman at a higher level of assertiveness takes charge of her life. She operates from an internal locus of control. She makes decisions. She takes chances. She acts instead of reacts.

When conflict arises, she sees it as potentially positive and actually enjoys challenges. Willingly she takes responsibility for her actions and their consequences. She makes significant choices and leaves little to chance.

Hardworking, energetic, and self-reliant, she radiates confidence. Although she is comfortable saying no, she delights in saying yes. In contrast to the first-level woman who "makes do" and the second-level woman who "won't do," her motto is "Can do!"

Beyond assertiveness. Just as the transition from remedial to basic assertiveness is long and difficult, getting from basic to advanced assertiveness requires another quantum jump. Once at the advanced level, however, it is merely a gradual slide into the fourth level. Perhaps "beyond assertiveness" is more of an extension than a level of its own.

At this point the woman incorporates all the attributes, attitudes, and actions previously discussed and more. High self-esteem is vital, but so is high esteem for others. The woman at this level is a powerful person in the most positive sense of the word. A high achiever in her own right, she also *enables* others to do their best work by maximizing their strengths instead of lingering on their limitations. Encounters with her leave others energized, not drained.

Positive and adventurous in her approach, the woman of beyond assertiveness is willing to take risks both personally and professionally. She not only chooses from alternatives, she also invents them. She creates jobs, markets, products, solutions, manuscripts. Innovation is her hallmark.

Her planning includes her lifetime and beyond. Much of what she is working on or for will benefit her children, grandchildren, and great-grandchildren. She is continually formulating, updating, redefining, and prioritizing her goals.

· · ·

As you consider these four levels of assertiveness, try to identify the level at which you entered the continuum, the level you have attained, and the level you would like to master. Are you growing in assertiveness or just thrashing around?

Don't be impatient. The metamorphosis from chicken to eagle takes time. If you are not quite ready to leave the barnyard for the mountaintop, at least hop on top of the chicken coop and see what is going on around you.

It may be lonely at the top, but it's crowded at the bottom. With each technical advance and each new service or pseudoservice, more and more people enter the health care industry: planners, evaluators, advisers, purchasers, programmers, assistants to assistants to assistants. Of course, the salary for each must be absorbed by the patients, even though the patients themselves may never benefit one iota. The burgeoning care payroll has no correlation with the quality or quantity of patient care given.

There may be some similarities between your hospital and a nationally known laboratory that had the habit of plotting the growth of the organization graphically each year. Two graphs were used: one for the administrative staff and one for the scientific and technological staff. Soon it became obvious that the administration had nearly tripled, whereas the number of scientists and technicians had remained almost constant. The solution was simple. Instead of cutting back on pencil pushers and red-tape worms or increasing the number of people actually doing the work, they simply opted to combine the graphs. Now the growth of the laboratory spirals ever upward, without making the proliferation of personnel parasites obvious.

A case in point may be one of the more recent positions to open up in the health care field: that of "patient advocate." First there was the token black, then the token woman, and now there's the token advocate. A lone individual, no matter how gifted or talented, cannot do what all of us who have vowed to serve and protect the patient cannot do. The existence of such a position provides false reassurance that the responsibility to stand up for the patient is no longer ours. "It's not my job, man. Let the advocate do it."

Much of the barnyard odor stems from the campaign to camouflage an inefficiently run industry as a charitable service. Health care is big business, and for women big business is still virtually off limits. To put business in a proper perspective, read *Up the Organization,* and *Further Up the Organization,* the best-selling books by Robert Townsend. In very humorous, readable form, Townsend outlines business problems and solutions, many of which are applicable to the health professions today. He is daring, imaginative, irreverent, and thoroughly practical. If he could do for the health care industry what he did for Avis Rent-a-Car, being a professional or a patient would be more profitable and pleasurable.

If you are involved in management at any level, you will find his theories on people and work, including everything from memos to mistresses, not only entertaining but useful. Townsend is unorthodox enough to suggest abolishing whole departments, such as purchasing, personnel, and public relations. He calls job descriptions "straitjackets" and boldly proposes making everyone stand up through some meetings to make sure they are mercifully short.

Meetings are a trademark of bureaucratic barnyards. How many times have you left a meeting feeling good about what you have accomplished, and how many times have you left feeling that your time has been totally wasted? Health professionals complain that they spend so much time in meetings talking about what should be done that there is no time left to do it.

If you share these feelings, check your calendar and appointment book. Are you attending meetings because *everyone* else does? Are you afraid of offending Big Daddy or Big Momma? Evaluate each meeting in light of the question: **Is what I am doing or about to do in the best interest of the patient?** Think of all the work that could be accomplished if *everyone* refused to attend meetings, refused to get bogged down in rhetoric, and finally admitted that hot air was getting us nowhere.

To further whet your appetite for Townsend's *Up the Organization*, here is an entire chapter titled "Excellence: Or What the Hell Are You Doing Here?": "If you don't do it excellently, don't do it at all. Because if it's not excellent it won't be profitable or fun, and if you're not in business for fun or profit, what the hell are you doing here?"*

Perhaps the time has come for you to ask yourself that question. What the hell are you doing in the health professions? If you work under conditions that do not permit you to do your work excellently, if the fun has gone out of your job, if it has not proved profitable for you or your patient, something is very wrong.

To right that wrong, you must first figure out what or who (self included) is keeping you from doing your work excellently. What obstacles stand between you and fun or profit?

---

*From Townsend R: *Up the Organization*, New York, 1970, Alfred A. Knopf.

If professionals do not receive satisfaction from their jobs, chances are neither will their patients. There are certain ingredients essential to job satisfaction. It does not matter whether a worker chooses to be a ditch digger, dietitian, bubble dancer, or doctor. Any worker's needs are basically these: belonging to a group, recognition, new experiences, and security.

Belonging to a group. Feelings of aloneness and isolation keep many women (especially housewives) from enjoying their jobs. No time to socialize and no one to socialize with are common complaints.

Within the health professions, work has become so specialized, so departmentalized and compartmentalized, that many of us feel a loneliness and isolation similar to that of housewives. Part-time workers and "floats" rarely feel they belong. Some express feeling like a visitor, an intruder, or a fifth wheel. Knowing that you are wanted, that you are welcome, that you belong is crucial to job satisfaction.

Even though your basic identity and strongest ties are wrapped up in family, you need a professional support group. You need colleagues with whom you can share both your joys and your sorrows. You need people around you who understand and care about you and your work, people who share some of your experiences, dreams, fears, priorities, and goals.

Women still have a lot to learn about teamwork, camaraderie, fellowship, and esprit de corps. Anything you can do to foster a one-for-all-and-all-for-one feeling, to give yourself and your colleagues a sense of belonging, a strong sense of "our" unit (hospital, agency, clients), will increase job satisfaction.

Recognition. Women and women's work are often taken for granted. If you are hungry for recognition, most likely the women around you feel the same way. You may all feel uncared for, unappreciated, and unnoticed. How long has it been since you told someone, "Hey, I really like working with you!"

It is nice to get praise from high places—the head of the hospital, the chief surgeon, the director of nurses—but for now perhaps we should work on recognizing each other. Sincere compliments, acknowledgments of jobs well done, a simple "thank you" can work wonders when it comes to job satisfaction. Use concrete phrases like "You are skillful with your hands" or "I admire the way you are able to organize your work" or "You certainly had a calming influence during that crisis" or "I feel confident when I have you as a team member."

Don't wait until a person retires or moves away to tell her how much she is appreciated. Every ego needs an occasional stroke for survival. That goes for doctors, head nurses, teachers, supervisors, and national leaders. If compliments were as quick and as bountiful as criticism, job satisfaction would increase immeasurably.

New experiences. For job satisfaction, it is essential to know the difference between specialization and stagnation. Everyone needs some variety, change, and challenge to keep growing. To shake things up, to keep awake and alert, try changing units, shifts, hospitals. Read! Attend a workshop. Take a class, even if it is in crochet. If you are community based, do a stint in the hospital; if hospital based, do a stint in the community.

There is no question that the health professions are demanding physically, mentally, and emotionally. Many of our jobs require great stamina and brute strength, since they involve bending, lifting, pulling, stretching, twisting, climbing, running, and being on our feet all day long. Add to the physical demands the emotional stress of being responsible for people who may be suffering or dying. Care, worry, sorrow, frustration, disappointment—all take their toll.

As you soak your feet, thankful just to have made it through another day, there is little energy left to reflect, plan, dream, or solve problems. Daily pressures, duties, and demands all crowd out the loftier, more noble goals you may have had when you first entered your profession.

Being ground-bound makes it difficult to get much perspective on the past, present, or future of the health care system. It makes it difficult to see beyond your own day-to-day work situation. You need some distance between yourself and the frenzied flock, a better vantage point from which to view problems and effect solutions.

One idea might be to work out an exchange program in which nurses, therapists, or social workers in the field change places with their counterparts in education every couple of years. Being on the front line would give educators an opportunity to get back to basics, to experience the problems encountered each day, and to try theories out in actual situations. Having workers move into the classroom would give students firsthand knowledge of life in the real world, with all its problems and pleasures. The workers could take some time to read, plan, and reflect before going back into practice.

When looking for new experiences, be sure to evaluate their relevance for you as an individual. Women health professionals have a history of feeling complimented when administration or medicine ordains us capable of absorbing some mundane task that they no longer desire to do. Women already do far more than our share of the world's menial tasks. Scut work seldom qualifies as a stimulating new experience.

Security. Certainly, security involves salary, fringe benefits, and pension plans, but it includes much more. Security means some type of predictability in the job and its demands. It means having some control over our professional environment. "Social security" should be extended to include not being subject to the whims, tirades, or vindictiveness of others and not being desperate to please superiors. Security means having a sense of worth, confidence, and respect.

·　　·　　·

If you are not deriving much satisfaction from your job, perhaps you can see whether a problem of belonging, recognition, new experiences, or security is giving you the most difficulty. Do not be discouraged if you find your professional life lacking in all four areas. Just as you learned to tackle one turkey at a time, tackle one area at a time. Start small, and be persistent. Remember that assertiveness is goal-oriented. You have to know what you want. As you perch atop the chicken coop, take time to assess where you've been, where you are, and where you would like to be.

Setting personal or professional goals is highly individual. To be a winner in life's game, you have to decide what "winning" is for you. Too many women are tempted to play by rules or for prizes that appeal to others. One woman's success is often another woman's failure.

Men and women have definite differences when it comes to defining "winners." It is fascinating to see how unsynchronized men's and women's needs and goals are at the same ages in life. If you thought growth and development stopped at age 18, read *Passages* by Gail Sheehy. Chapters such as "Why Can't a Woman Be More Like a Man and a Man Be Less Like a Racehorse?" help explain, comfort, and encourage those of us who find we are still having growing pains in our middle and later years. As you approach assertiveness, it will make a difference whether you are in your twenties, thirties, forties, or fifties. *Passages* will help women and men who are sick of barnyard mentality but afraid of heights to dare venture up to the mountaintop. The book may also help you avoid a trap that many women have fallen into—that of mimicking men.

Although it is true that men have it better than women in almost every sphere, being masculine in your desires, attitudes, or actions will not make you an optimum human being. It is as unhealthy and unproductive for women to adopt the male model as it is for women health professionals to adopt the medical model. Men's rules and men's prizes rarely have relevance for women. Under these circumstances, even women who are winners feel like losers.

Another trouble spot for men and women is the dependence-independence-interdependence spiral. It is supposed that each level represents one more step toward maturity. In our culture, however, men have been allowed—and encouraged—to occupy the independent level as their own. Women, who rarely taste independence, split their lives between the dependent and interdependent levels, resulting in a splitting headache.

We go from being dependent on our parents to being depended on by husbands and children. We are cared for and then suddenly jump to caring for others without ever really learning how to care for ourselves. It is almost as though women have missed a step and stumbled into maturity without recognizing it. Conflict and confusion arise because although women may have arrived on the interdependent plateau in interpersonal relationships, we are still very dependent on men economically and politically. Our blatant dependence in these areas tends to obscure our interdependence in other areas.

Serving others is an interdependent function. However, those who are self-serving view it as a dependent function. Once again, it becomes critical to find a way of serving others without being subservient.

Much of the shame, anger, and unrest women are experiencing results from the mislabeling of our functions as dependent and the failure of both men and women to recognize these functions as interdependent. Although it is expedient for women to strive for more independence in economic and political situations, it would be disastrous for us to deny ourselves the social and emotional interdependence that we have already achieved.

Women have a working knowledge of interdependence. We understand and accept needing, feeling, giving, compromising, placing others first, sharing, and caring. We have firsthand knowledge of the cost in time and energy that is required to sustain and nurture other human beings. Yet each day, men who have far less experience and insight into these matters designate priorities and formulate policies that regulate birth, death, and everything in between.

Although it may be true that women do not know much about looking out for Number One, we know a great deal about looking out for others. If there is one area in which women excel, it is caregiving. This is why it is so unfortunate that women are excluded from the decision-making processes that regulate the who, what, when, where, why, and how of caregiving systems.

Watching congressional debates on abortion issues is a visual reminder of how women are excluded from decisions that uniquely and profoundly affect us. Although our elected officials may be able to legislate that a woman give life to a baby, they cannot legislate that she give love. Sadly, unwanted children too often grow up into unwanted adults. The eventual cost of uncared for and poorly cared for children may really be staggering.

Although it is exhilarating to snatch a fetus or a felon from the jaws of death, that brief act sets years of caregiving in motion. The flash of medical or legal brilliance dims quickly, and the men move on to new conquests, while women move in to mop up. Over the years, women health professionals have spent much of their time caring for the living remains of legal and medical miracles. Men are too busy to salvage and sustain. Perhaps if they were required to share in these functions, they would come to the realization that death is not the worst thing that can happen to a human being.

But for now, salvaging and sustaining are women's work. Unless women in the health professions learn to speak up and stand up for the rights of humans, atrocities like the following will continue indefinitely.

Whatever happened to the Old West tradition of letting people die with their boots on? Today we won't even let them die with their feet on. Not too many years ago, the Supreme Court rejected the pleas of 72-year-old Mary Northern of Nashville, Tennessee, to prevent doctors from amputating her gangrenous feet. Lawyers for the "elderly recluse" said she had a "right to privacy" and a fundamental right of "bodily integrity." They observed that no lower court had ruled her incompetent for any purpose other than deciding whether she needed this particular operation.

According to her lawyers, Mary had only a 5 to 10 percent chance of survival without the amputation and about a 50 percent chance of survival with it. Given only a fifty-fifty chance of survival, the will to live often tips the balance. Just a few years ago, a similar case received national attention. Another elderly woman had her leg amputated against her will. She died a few weeks after the operation.

If Mary Northern survived the surgery, what would her life be like?

A woman who has lived alone for 17 years, suddenly denied her privacy, freedom, and independence. Consigned to a "businessing" or "doctoring" home or parking lot (formerly known as "nursing home") to await death. If you were forced to have such mutilating surgery against your will at the age of 72, how long do you think you would survive?

Perhaps it is not the function of physicians or state officials or Supreme Court justices to consider such things. But someone should consider such things. Perhaps the assertive thing for women in the health professions to do would be to form a humane society for humans. Animals should not be the only ones protected from torture and mutilation.

Angels of mercy or accomplices to crime? You be the judge after reading about the following timeless description of life in the health care barnyard, vividly depicted in an article by Priscilla Johnson called "The Long, Hard Dying of Joe Rodriguez" (*American Journal of Nursing*, January 1977). She describes a nightmare situation involving a heroin addict who has been stabbed in the abdomen. He arrives on the intensive care unit from surgery still hemorrhaging, on a respirator, and with his entire pancreas and colon hopelessly necrotic. Not expected to live through the night, he manages to survive several days.

Joe is surrounded by machines, his body punctured with a dozen tubes. His care is laborious and mechanical. The physicians concentrate on tissues, organs, fluids, and electrolytes, apparently unable to see the forest for the trees.

A week after his admission, he hemorrhages, his gut falls out, and they race him to surgery doing CPR all the way. Somehow he survives surgery but is soon hemorrhaging again. The blood bank is screaming because it is bankrupt. The stench, the pain, the degradation, the futility are all explicitly detailed.

When the author leaves the room for a few minutes, she hears the angry reactions of women who question the terrible waste of blood, sweat, and tears. They plead to let him go. Everyone seems to agree that what they are doing is wrong, everyone but the medical staff.

A new intern enters the case, telling the author that Joe's problem is reversible, that he can improve. Silently she questions: "Sir, do you really mean it? You're actually telling me that Joe will someday walk out of here—leaving his pancreas, his kidneys, his bowels behind? Is what they have told you true, or is it only that the insatiable vanity of the medical team will not admit defeat?"

Throughout the ordeal, the recurring question she asks herself is:

"What is right, what is really loving Joe Rodriguez?" It is a question she does not ask aloud, because, as she says, "That question just doesn't seem to matter."

As she describes the situation, that question does not appear to matter to the medical staff, but it seems to matter a great deal to the nurses. Among themselves, they agonize over the standing order to resuscitate Joe Rodriguez. They question and cry, but they stop short of confronting the medical staff with their concerns and convictions.

Unfortunately, the Joe Rodriguez situation is not that uncommon. Most women in the health professions have a horror story or two to match this one. The time has come for women to loudly ask what is right, what is the loving thing to do. Women may be in a better position than men to assess whether life is being sustained or death is being prolonged.

Ostriches, get your heads out of the sand! These are only samples of the hard issues that need to be grappled with in the health professions, and they will not go away if ignored. The consequences of action or inaction are fearful. There are no simple solutions, no pat formulas for instant success. Assertiveness is not a cure-all. It is only a first step. But watch that first step; it's a long one.

Although the problems in health care may be bigger than both of us, they are not bigger than all of us. If women win the right to share equally with men in making life-and-death decisions, our rewards will be greater but so will our responsibilities. If you are too chicken to share those responsibilities, you had better begin again at page 1. If you are too tired or too timid to share the load, then pass your proxy to those who can. Let local and national leaders in political and professional organizations know where you stand on the tough issues.

The assertive response is basically to ask yourself: "What can *I* do? What can I do right *now*?" And then do it.

Two must-read books that capture the struggle of women caught somewhere between the barnyard and the mountaintop are *Megatrends for Women* and *Backlash*. If you want to get high, read *Megatrends for Women,* authored by the same dynamic duo, Patricia Aburdene and John Naisbitt, that brought us the best-sellers *Megatrends* and *Megatrends 2000*. Their theory is that women are about to reach "critical mass" in politics, business, sports, religion, and more. Critical mass, a theory borrowed from physics, is the point at which a process becomes self-sustaining. The metaphor they use is an avalanche. One by one, women have fought for acceptance and achievement on this planet. They see women poised on the brink, about to be swept into success, with a force that will literally be "unstoppable." It is exhilarating reading.

To bring you back down to earth, read *Backlash: The Undeclared War Against American Women.* Pulitzer Prize–winning journalist Susan Faludi chronicles the rise and fall of the women's movement in the past 100 years. Whenever women seem be attaining critical mass, a backlash develops to keep women "in their place."

Faludi does not bring us the *bad* news. She brings us the *real* news. She thoroughly documents how "facts" presented in today's news stories are mostly fiction. There is no man shortage, there is no infertility epidemic, and high-powered, successful women are not fleeing the workplace to return to domestic bliss. It is a hoax. And it is part of a backlash designed to take away the minimal progress women have made in politics, business, sports, religion, and more.

Aburdene and Naisbitt caution us that critical mass for women has not yet come and that it will not be enough. Women must use the energy of critical mass to take appropriate action. They see sabotage as a possibility. Faludi sees it as reality. After reading *Backlash,* you will question what you see in the news, what you read in "scientific" journals, what you hear in sermons or political speeches, what you view in the movie theater, and what the fashion industry tries to dictate.

Since women constitute 80 to 85 percent of all health care workers, it would appear we reached critical mass in health care years ago and several times over. Yet we still lack clout when it comes to critical issues. Assertiveness is one way to energize, activate, and achieve our potential.

There will be days when you will wish you had never heard of assertiveness, days when you wish you could just fly away and not have to toil in the health care barnyard. There will be days when you won't quite know who you are or what your place is. There will be days when things seem to stand still or, worse yet, days when you are sure things are moving backward. Take heart. Those days are numbered.

On days when you feel all alone in the universe, get out and look for birds of a feather. Take the initiative to share some of what you are going through with others, and they may open up and share with you. Some may even dare join you if they know where you are going.

Keep your eye on the center—the patient. Focus on the patient, and you will be amazed at how the petty, peripheral things will float away, and your work will seem less complicated and cluttered.

Hunt and peck and scratch and claw, but take time to dream. Be prepared for some highs and lows, knowing that you are bound to win some and lose some. Know that nothing or no one is forever. Learn to let go of everything except your sense of humor.

Each reader will have to write her own epilogue. For now, here is a benediction:

> But they that wait upon the Lord shall renew their strength: they shall mount up with wings as eagles: they shall run, and not be weary: and they shall walk, and not faint. (Isaiah 40:31)

Ready for lift-off? Then straighten up and fly . . . right?

Annotated bibliography

Aburdene, Patricia, and Naisbitt, John: *Megatrends for Women,* New York, 1992, Villard Books.

An optimistic, visionary look at how women are leading a revolution in everything from sports to religion, business to politics. The authors see women as the key to solving some of society's most intractable problems, from homelessness to environmental concerns.

Ailes, Roger: *You Are the Message,* New York, 1988, Doubleday.

Seven seconds. That's all you have to communicate who and what you are. Ailes, who advises top executives, celebrities, and politicians, tells how to get your message across whether you are addressing 2 people or 2000. Eye-opening advice on verbal and nonverbal communication skills.

Alberti, Robert E., and Emmons, Michael L.: *Your Perfect Right: A Guide to Assertive Behavior,* San Luis Obispo, Calif., 1970, Impact Series.

A pioneer effort in assertiveness training. Aims to enrich the humanity of all by increasing the self-esteem in each of us. Gives multiple case examples with conclusions to illustrate assertive, nonassertive, and aggressive behavior. Contains a step-by-step outline for asserting yourself, along with a guide to becoming a therapist and helping others become more assertive. Includes annotated bibliography.

Alberti, Robert E., and Emmons, Michael L.: *Stand Up, Speak Out, Talk Back!* New York, 1975, Pocket Books.

After reading this book, many women feel they should have its title embossed on their T-shirts. Loaded with practical examples for social, school, and work situations. Contains tips on forming an assertiveness training group and on helping others learn to be assertive.

Armstrong, Alexandra, and Donahue, Mary R.: *On Your Own: A Widow's Passage to Emotional & Financial Well-Being,* 1993, Dearborn Financial Publishing, Inc.

A certified financial planner and a psychologist team up to provide a practical, compassionate guide for helping women deal with the emotional, as well as the financial, consequences of widowhood. An absolutely excellent resource.

Baer, Jean: *How to Be an Assertive (Not Aggressive) Woman in Life, in Love, and on the Job,* New York, 1976, New American Library.

After a lifetime of "dependency training," the author encourages women to seek assertiveness training. Contains well-written, thoroughly documented, detailed case studies, including interviews with several highly successful women. Tells how to spot your own blocks to assertiveness and gives exercises to overcome them. Emphasizes assertiveness in close relationships, as well as on the job. Contains an entire chapter on children and assertiveness.

Beattie, Melody: *Codependent No More: How to Stop Controlling Others and Start Caring for Yourself,* New York, 1987, Harper/Hazelden.

More than you ever wanted to know about codependence. She not only wrote the books, she lived them. Fascinating. Helpful. For those of us in health care, codependence is an occupational hazard. Also by the author: *Beyond Codependency* (New York, 1989, Harper/Hazelden) and *Codependent's Guide to the Twelve Steps* (New York, 1990, Prentice Hall).

Caplan, Paula J.: *The Myth of Women's Masochism,* New York, 1987, Signet.

Debunks the myth that women are inherently masochistic and have an innate need to suffer. This widespread view that some men have, allowing them to blame the victim, can permanently delay correcting the social institutions that are primary causes of the trouble. Examines why women are attracted to men who abuse them, why mothers are always blamed for children's problems, how "therapists" may be doing much more harm for women than good, and much more.

Carter-Scott, Cherie: *The Corporate Negaholic: How to Successfully Deal with Negative Colleagues, Managers, and Corporations,* New York, 1991, Villard Books.

If you've ever thought your organization was sick, you will find "the ten characteristics of dysfunctional companies" fascinating. The author colorfully describes negative individuals, departments, and corporations and then prescribes effective actions. If you are part of the problem, the final chapter deals with self-management.

Covey, Stephen R.: *The Seven Habits of Highly Effective People,* New York, 1990, Simon & Schuster.

Best-seller that encourages all of us to move from dependence through independence to interdependence. Covey defines habits as "the intersection of knowledge, skill, and desire." The seven habits are (1) be proactive; (2) begin with the end in mind; (3) put first things first; (4) think win/win; (5) seek first to understand . . . then to be understood; (6) synergize; and (7) sharpen the saw—which means taking care of yourself physically, mentally, spiritually, and emotionally. If you like this one, check out *Principled-Centered Leadership* (New York, 1992, Simon & Schuster) by the same author.

Cowan, Connell, and Kinder, Melvyn: *Smart Women: Foolish Choices,* New York, 1985, Clarkson N. Potter.

Best-seller that examines why women not only settle for men who are not their equal, but actually tend to seek them out. Being foolish includes searching for the perfect man, needing to be rescued, refusing to grow up, and being attracted to men who make miserable partners. Getting smart means breaking the addiction to love and romance, investing in long-term relationships, and making choices.

Ellis, Albert, and Hunter, Patricia A.: *Why Am I Always Broke? How to Be Sane About Money,* New York, 1991, Carol Publishing Group.

Stop making yourself crazy when it comes to money! Written by the founder of rational-emotive therapy, this book shows how to deprogram yourself, whether you spend too little or too much. Helps you examine and change your basic attitudes and actions when it comes to money. You'll want to pay special attention to Chapter 7: "Being Female and Financially Savvy: Women and Managing Money."

Faludi, Susan: *Backlash: The Undeclared War Against American Women,* New York, 1991, Crown.

This Pulitzer Prize–winning author thoroughly documents how women's minimal progress in business and politics is being actively sabotaged. *Backlash* will make you question what you read in "scientific" journals and realize that "news" stories are often more fiction than fact. What you see on TV, at the movies, and in the fashion magazines will confirm there is an "undeclared war against American women."

Fensterheim, Herbert: *Don't Say Yes When You Want to Say No,* New York, 1975, Dell.
  Gives a strong theoretical background linking assertiveness training with behavior therapy. Includes an assertiveness inventory; instructions for setting goals and achieving them (for instance, how to get thin and stay thin); and suggestions for handling social situations, sexual relationships, habits, depression, and assertiveness on the job. Excellent case examples and some personal sharing by the author.

Fournies, Ferdinand F.: *Why Employees Don't Do What They're Supposed to Do and What to Do About It,* New York, 1988, Liberty Hall Press.
  A quick read. Practical tips on how to improve performance and get results from people working with you or for you. *Why* don't people do what they are supposed to do? Myriad reasons, including not knowing how to do it, thinking their way is better, having no reward or possibly being punished for doing it, personal limits, impossible tasks, and more. Each chapter describes a problem and then gives a preventive solution.

Harris, Thomas A.: *I'm Ok—You're Ok: A Practical Guide to Transactional Analysis,* New York, 1967, Harper & Row.
  Excellent reading for those who want to explore transactional analysis in more detail. Clear presentation of the Parent, Adult, and Child in all of us. Gives practical situations and solutions for times when communication becomes snarled and tangled. Contains interesting chapters on moral values, social implications, and family interactions.

Harvey, Joan C.: *If I'm So Successful, Why Do I Feel Like a Fake? The Impostor Phenomenon,* New York, 1985, Pocket Books.
  Do you think you have fooled other people into overestimating your ability? Do you attribute your success to some factor other than intelligence or ability? Do you fear being exposed as a fraud? If you answered yes to all three of these questions, you are a victim of the Impostor Phenomenon. The IP is related to but different from self-esteem issues. This book is especially recommended for those of you leaving comfortable clinical roles and moving into administration, academia, or other roles of authority and autonomy. Contains the Harvey IP Scale tĬhat you can use to assess the degree to which the IP might be affecting your personal or professional life. Includes information on how this phenomenon develops; how it influences the way you think, feel, and act; and finally how to free yourself from its debilitating effects.

Henning, Margaret, and Jardim, Anne: The *Managerial Woman,* New York, 1977, Pocket Books.
  Excellently written by two women with doctoral degrees from Harvard Business School. Although based on their work with women managers in the business world, the book has endless implications for working women everywhere. Intelligent, helpful view of the real world, not the ideal world. Explains differences between men and women regarding upbringing, expectations, opportunities, career choices, and constraints. Must reading for the professional woman seeking a career, not just a string of jobs.

Hewlett, Sylvia Ann: *A Lesser Life: The Myth of Women's Liberation in America,* New York, 1986, Warner Books.
  Thoroughly researched and impeccably documented. Filled with eye-opening case histories and touching personal examples. Demonstrates American women's immense economic vulnerability and why no matter how well-educated, talented, or hard-working a woman may be, her career will be "sabotaged by motherhood." Learn how far our country's day care, parental leave, and other social support systems lag behind other industrialized civilizations. READ THIS BOOK!

Hirsch, Gretchen: *Womanhours: A 21 Day Time Management Plan That Works,* New York, 1983, St. Martins Press.
  Discusses the bind women are in trying to conform to a double standard that requires

them to be basically passive yet quick-witted, strong, and resourceful. Suggests women do not need tips on how to cram more into their tight schedules but a system that lets them choose whose needs they will respond to. ("Efficiency doesn't breed happiness, effectiveness does.") Loaded with practical advice on keeping time logs, stripping away unnecessary tasks, clearing up role confusion, and positive planning.

Hochschild, Arlie: *The Second Shift: Working Parents and the Revolution at Home,* New York, 1989, Viking.

Surprise, surprise—there seems to be a 15-hour-per-week leisure gap between men and women. Despite all the talk of shared parenting and household chores, women continue to work a "second shift." After following 10 couples over an 8-year period, the author provides both philosophical and practical information on how two-paycheck families can better cope with overextended lives.

Huseman, Richard C., and Hatfield, John D.: *Managing the Equity Factor . . . or 'After All I've Done for You . . .',* Boston, 1989, Houghton Mifflin.

Designed for managers but applicable to all of us as we struggle for healthy relationships. Trouble begins when there is a "perceived" lack of balance or equity between what we get and what we give. (Facts don't count. Perception is everything.) Power lies in positive expectations, goal setting, performance feedback, and what they call novel, rewarding behavior. Good on the job and off.

Jongeward, Dorothy, and Scott, Dru: *Women As Winners: Transactional Analysis for Personal Growth,* Reading, Mass., 1979, Addison-Wesley.

A practical, positive book that draws on transactional analysis, Gestalt therapy, and life scripting to help women understand the past, survive the present, and succeed in the future. Explodes most of the myths and fairy tales women have unthinkingly embraced. Documents the harsh financial realities most women must face.

Jongeward, Dorothy, and Seyer, Philip: *Choosing Success: Transactional Analysis on the Job,* New York, 1978, John Wiley & Sons.

For *STAT* readers interested in learning more about transactional analysis, this is an excellent book. The first half deals with TA on the job, and the second half focuses on one's personal life. Each chapter begins with objectives, ends with a summary, and is chock full of examples, exercises, flowcharts, and illustrations. Whether you are a worker or a working supervisor, you will appreciate practical tips on such things as how to assertively disagree, how to manage your time, and how to confront people (subordinates, superiors, peers, and clients) in a straight forward manner.

Jorgensen, James: *How to Stay Ahead in the Money Game,* New York, 1986, Stein & Day.

Part One explains what financial deregulation means to personal money management and how clinging to old money habits may mean losing 20 percent of your income each year. Part Two is filled with practical tips for the building years (30-45), the middle years (45-60), and the retirement years (60 plus). Solid advice for financial planning based on your goals and your personality. Contains a glossary of economic and investment terms, as well as the names and addresses of organizations where you can get additional information and help.

Kaminer, Wendy: *I'm Dysfunctional—You're Dysfunctional,* Reading, Mass., 1992, Addison-Wesley.

Skeptical of the self-help movement? Read this critique of America's "recovery" obsession in which people have begun to pride themselves on being immature, addicted, and dysfunctional. Far from being "self-help," this billion-dollar-a-year industry encourages passivity, conformity, and stupidity.

Laut, Phil: *Money Is My Friend,* New York, 1989, Ivy Books.

Bizarre, yet fascinating, approach to gaining financial freedom. Evidently, most of us have a poverty, not a prosperity, mentality. Explodes myths about money and suggests that until you make friends with it, you will never amass much of it. Includes four laws of wealth: the earning law, the spending law, the saving law, and the investing law.

Melia, Jinx, and Lyttle, Pauline: *Why Jenny Can't Lead: Understanding the Male Dominant System,* Grand Junction, Colo., 1986, Operational Politics.

Documents how women continue to misread and mishandle power from historical times to the present. Teaches women how to accommodate to the world rather than expecting the world to accommodate them. Noting "there is almost nothing in this society controlled by women," the authors explain how to play politics on male turf. Includes learning to barter, negotiate, interpret, speak, behave, and become a good team player. Definitely a book for women with advanced assertiveness skills who continue to be puzzled by their lack of success.

Miller, Jean Baker: *Toward a New Psychology of Women,* Boston, 1976, Beacon Press.

If women's subordinate position in society has ever made you furious or depressed, this book will explain, comfort, and challenge you. Based on clinical observations, the author examines conflict, cooperation, and creativity, as well as other aspects of life. Miller sees within women strengths and insights that have been largely ignored. Invigorating glimpse into the future when both men and women can set aside rigid stereotypes and become fully human.

Moore, Lynda L.: *Not As Far As You Think: The Realities of Working Women,* Lexington, Mass., 1986, Lexington Press.

The title says it all.

Norwood, Robin: *Women Who Love Too Much,* New York, 1986, Pocket Books.

If your marriage seems to be an extension of your caseload, read this book. Sensitive, compassionate women are often drawn to unhealthy, unloving partners. Using powerful words like "obsession" and "addiction," the author gives numerous case studies that demonstrate how these relationships develop, deteriorate, and destroy the people involved. Contains a 10-point recovery plan guaranteed to work, BUT the author cautions that these "simple" steps will take years of total commitment to fully implement.

O'Reilly, Jane: *The Girl I Left Behind,* New York, 1980, Macmillan.

Subtitled *The Housewife's Moment of Truth and Other Feminist Ravings,* this book is a humorous, personal account of the people, places, and events that made the author a feminist (a person—man or woman—who makes a conscious and continuous effort to improve the lives of all women). As a journalist, O'Reilly discovered that the same problems face women all over the world: inadequate education, low wages, lack of political power, legal inequality, denial of control over their own bodies. Eventually, she discovered to her surprise that as a woman they were *her* problems, too.

Porter, Sylvia: *Love & Money,* New York, 1985, William Morrow.

Frank discussions about financial planning whether you are single, widowed, divorced, cohabiting, or even a mistress. Loaded with case studies and budget makeovers. Realistic money management for today's shifting relationships.

Rivers, Caryl, Barnett, Rosalind, and Baruch, Grace: *Beyond Sugar and Spice: How Women Grow, Learn, and Thrive,* New York, 1979, Ballantine Books.

Absolutely crammed with facts, figures, and personal and professional insights to help women understand their lives. If you have a daughter, this book will help you provide her

STAT

with self-confidence, resourcefulness, and the general ability to take care of herself. Highly recommended.

Shaevitz, Marjorie Hansen: *The Superwoman Syndrome,* New York, 1984, Warner Books.
Explores the physical and psychological effects of being overworked and overstressed. Contains a comprehensive questionnaire to help you pinpoint your individual problems. Teaches how to deal with a traditional feminine upbringing in today's world, including everything from improving relationships to how and why you can and should do *less* housework. Includes a chapter by her husband, psychologist Morton H. Shaevitz, titled "How Men Really Feel" (about home, children, sex, and working wives).

Sheehy, Gail: *Passages: Predictable Crises of Adult Life,* New York, 1974, E.P. Dutton.
Must reading for any woman between the ages of 20 and 50. Most of us in the health professions have studied child growth and development. We have mistakenly concluded that this process ends with adolescence. It is reassuring and exciting to know that growth and change continue throughout life and that adult stages are as distinct, as fascinating, as painful, and as promising as any of the childhood stages. Especially helpful in understanding that men and women experience different stages at different ages.

Sheehy, Gail: *Pathfinders,* New York, 1981, William Morrow.
If you relished *Passages,* you will delight in *Pathfinders* even more. Pathfinders are not charmed human beings but ordinary people from all age groups and all walks of life who have faced a crisis in an unusually creative way. The emphasis is on well-being, a state achieved by these people who were not afraid to take risks or make changes in their lives.

Smith, Manuel J.: *When I Say No I Feel Guilty,* New York, 1975, Dial Press.
Extensive dialogues used to illustrate a variety of assertive techniques. Situations range from your bedroom to your place of business. If you are confused about what assertive speech sounds like, Smith offers abundant examples. He also provides a list of rights, including your right to say, "I don't care."

Tannen, Deborah: *You Just Don't Understand: Women and Men in Conversation,* New York, 1990, Ballantine Books.
Tannen's first book—*That's Not What I Meant!*—focused on communication differences spawned by geographic, ethnic, or class backgrounds. This one focuses on gender differences. Men and women come from vastly different cultures. We do not speak the same language. For example, when a woman says, "I'm sorry," she is expressing concern. When a man hears "I'm sorry," he thinks you are assuming blame. It's a miracle we can work together, let alone live together!

Van Caspel, Venita: *The Power of Money Dynamics,* Reston, Va., 1983, Reston.
If you are only going to read one book on money management, make it this one. Unravels the mysteries of the world of high finance and points the way to financial independence. Contains everything from how to read a prospectus to how to bankroll a college education. Includes a chapter on life insurance that reveals that most of us are paying way too much and few of us even have the right kind of policy.